KT-384-855

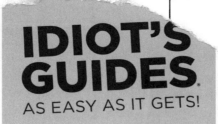

IDIOT'S GUIDES.
AS EASY AS IT GETS!

The Mediterranean Diet Cookbook

by Denise "DedeMed" Hazime

ALPHA

ALPHA BOOKS

Published by Penguin Group (USA) Inc.

Penguin Group (USA) Inc., 375 Hudson Street, New York, New York 10014, USA • Penguin Group (Canada), 90 Eglinton Avenue East, Suite 700, Toronto, Ontario M4P 2Y3, Canada (a division of Pearson Penguin Canada Inc.) • Penguin Books Ltd., 80 Strand, London WC2R 0RL, England • Penguin Ireland, 25 St. Stephen's Green, Dublin 2, Ireland (a division of Penguin Books Ltd.) • Penguin Group (Australia), 250 Camberwell Road, Camberwell, Victoria 3124, Australia (a division of Pearson Australia Group Pty. Ltd.) • Penguin Books India Pvt. Ltd., 11 Community Centre, Panchsheel Park, New Delhi—110 017, India • Penguin Group (NZ), 67 Apollo Drive, Rosedale, North Shore, Auckland 1311, New Zealand (a division of Pearson New Zealand Ltd.) • Penguin Books (South Africa) (Pty.) Ltd., 24 Sturdee Avenue, Rosebank, Johannesburg 2196, South Africa • Penguin Books Ltd., Registered Offices: 80 Strand, London WC2R 0RL, England

International Standard Book Number: 978-1-61564-445-2
Library of Congress Catalog Card Number: 2013956275

17 16 15 14   10 9 8 7 6 5 4 3 2 1

Interpretation of the printing code: The rightmost number of the first series of numbers is the year of the book's printing; the rightmost number of the second series of numbers is the number of the book's printing. For example, a printing code of 14-1 shows that the first printing occurred in 2014.

Printed in the United States of America

Note: This publication contains the opinions and ideas of its author. It is intended to provide helpful and informative material on the subject matter covered. It is sold with the understanding that the author and publisher are not engaged in rendering professional services in the book. If the reader requires personal assistance or advice, a competent professional should be consulted. The author and publisher specifically disclaim any responsibility for any liability, loss, or risk, personal or otherwise, which is incurred as a consequence, directly or indirectly, of the use and application of any of the contents of this book.

Most Alpha books are available at special quantity discounts for bulk purchases for sales promotions, premiums, fund-raising, or educational use. Special books, or book excerpts, can also be created to fit specific needs. For details, write: Special Markets, Alpha Books, 375 Hudson Street, New York, NY 10014.

Publisher: *Mike Sanders*
Executive Managing Editor: *Billy Fields*
Senior Acquisitions Editor: *Brook Farling*
Development Editorial Supervisor: *Christy Wagner*
Senior Production Editor: *Janette Lynn*

Cover Designer: *Laura Merriman*
Book Designer: *William Thomas*
Indexer: *Tonya Heard*
Layout: *Ayanna Lacey*
Proofreader: *Laura Caddell*

Contents

Part 1:   What the Mediterranean Diet's All About 1

1   What Is the Mediterranean Diet?............................3

A Little History...4

The Benefits of the Mediterranean Diet...4

Disease Prevention..4

Weight Loss...5

Superb Nutrition..6

Components of the Mediterranean Diet and Lifestyle.....................7

On the Menu: Fresh, Nutritious Food..8

Making Time for Exercise...9

Reducing Stress...9

Family Time...10

Eating Out on the Diet...10

Changing for the Better...10

2   The Mediterranean Kitchen 13

The Mediterranean Diet Pyramid..14

Mediterranean Foods and Ingredients...15

Fresh Fruits and Vegetables...16

Whole Grains..18

Legumes and Nuts...19

Meats, Poultry, and Eggs...20

Stocking Your Pantry...21

Spices and Herbs..21

Salt...22

Olive Oil...22

Cheese and Yogurt..23

Honey, Waters, and Syrups...23

Part 2:   Mediterranean Breakfasts and Brunches..............25

3   Quick Breakfasts...27

Yogurt Spread (Labne)..28

Yogurt Bowl..29

Quick Cream of Wheat..30

Garlic Scrambled Eggs...31

Holiday Eggs...32

Mediterranean Omelet...33

Potatoes and Eggs Omelet..34

Herbed Potatoes and Eggs...35

Fried Cheese..36

4   Brunch Bites...37

Breakfast Casserole (Fatteh)......................................38

Mediterranean Breakfast Quiche.................................39

Shanklish Cheese..40

Cheesy Breakfast Pizza (Cheese Manakish)..................41

Thyme Breakfast Pizza (Zaatar Manakish)..................42

Breakfast Beans (Ful Mudammas).............................43

Chicken Liver..44

Sweet Bread with Dates...45

Part 3:   Lunch on the Mediterranean 47

5   Lovely Lunch Salads 49

Tabbouleh Salad..50

Fattoush Salad..51

Mediterranean Garden Salad...................................52

Tomato and Cucumber Salad....................................53

Mediterranean Potato Salad.....................................54

Roasted Beet Salad..55

Quinoa Salad..56

Warm Mediterranean Salad.....................................57

Mediterranean Pasta Salad......................................58

Spinach Salad...59

Greek Salad..60

Lentil Salad..61

Bean Salad...62

Fig Salad..63

Watermelon Salad...64

Mediterranean Dressing..65

6   Super Soups...67

Beef and Vegetable Soup..68

Chicken Soup..69

Pumpkin Soup...70

Yellow Lentil Soup...71

Hearty Brown Lentil Soup..72

Lentil and Swiss Chard Soup *74*

Freekeh Soup *75*

Barley and Chicken Soup *76*

7   Soothing Stews **77**

Ghallaba Stew *78*

Eggplant Stew *79*

Jew's Mallow Stew (Mulukhiya) *80*

Okra Stew (Bamya) *81*

Green Pea Stew (Bazella) *82*

Cauliflower Stew *83*

Green Bean Stew *84*

8   Meaty Mediterranean Lunches **85**

Beefy Pita Sandwiches *86*

Kefta Burgers *87*

Baked Spaghetti with Beef *88*

Hearty Meat and Potatoes *89*

Beef-Stuffed Squash (Kusa Mihshi) *90*

Beef-Stuffed Baked Potatoes *91*

Lamb-Stuffed Baked Peppers *92*

Lamb Cabbage Rolls (Malfouf) *93*

Cheeseless Meat Pizza (Lahme bi Ajeen) *94*

Breaded Chicken (Chicken Escalope) *95*

Chicken Phyllo Rolls (Msakhan) *96*

Chicken Quinoa Pilaf *97*

Fish with Tahini Sauce (Fish Tagine) *98*

Lemon Cilantro Shrimp *99*

Grilled Shrimp Sandwiches with Pesto *100*

Shrimp and Vegetable Rice *101*

Basil and Shrimp Quinoa *102*

9   Very Vegetarian Lunches **103**

Falafel Pita Pockets *104*

Couscous with Vegetable Stew *105*

Sweet and Savory Couscous *106*

Macaroni with Yogurt Sauce *107*

Vegetable Grape Leaves *108*

Eggplant Casserole (Moussaka) *109*

Green Beans and Tomatoes *110*

Zucchini Fritters *111*

Spanakopita 112

Zesty Flatbread Pizza 113

Mediterranean Grilled Cheese Sandwiches 114

Fried Eggplant and Cauliflower Sandwiches 115

10   Great Grain, Rice, and Bean Dishes........................ 117

Bulgur with Seasoned Lamb 118

Bulgur Chickpea Pilaf 119

Bulgur Tomato Pilaf 120

Freekeh Pilaf 121

Spiced Tomato No-Bake Pilaf 122

Pumpkin Kibbeh 123

Zucchini and Brown Rice 124

*Lentils and Rice (*Mujaddara with Rice*)* 125

*Lentils and Bulgur Wheat Pilaf (*Mujaddara Hamra*)* 126

Part 4:   Snacks, Sauces, and More..127

11   Delightful Dips and Spreads 129

Traditional Hummus 130

Hummus with Meat 131

Cilantro Jalapeño Hummus 132

Roasted Red Pepper Hummus 133

White Bean Hummus 134

Volcano Feta 135

Muhammara *Spread* 136

*Eggplant Dip (*Mutabal*)* 137

Olive Tapenade 138

Roasted Red Pepper and Sun-Dried Tomato Tapenade 139

Baba Ganoush 140

12   Appealing Appetizers and Breads 141

Hummus Appetizer Bites 142

Aromatic Artichokes 143

Cheese Rolls 144

Spinach Pies 145

*Meat-Filled Phyllo (*Samboosek*)* 146

*Beef Tartar (*Kibbeh Nayeh*)* 147

Pita Bread 148

Savory Pita Chips 149

Rosemary Olive Bread 150

Multipurpose Dough 151

13   Sauces, Spices, and Condiments **153**

Tzatziki Sauce *154*

Homemade Greek Yogurt *155*

Tahini Paste *156*

*Tahini Sauce (*Tarator*)* *157*

Garlic Sauce *158*

Lemon Basil Garlic Sauce *159*

*Hot Sauce (*Harissa*)* *160*

Zaatar *161*

Seven Spice Mix *162*

Part 5:   Mouthwatering Mediterranean Mains **163**

14   Beef and Lamb Dinners **165**

Beef Shawarma *166*

Kefta Kabob *167*

Kibbeh with Yogurt *168*

Kibbeh in a Pan *169*

Beef Shish Kabobs *170*

Tomato and Beef Casserole *171*

*Upside-Down Rice (*Makloubeh*)* *172*

Meat and Rice–Stuffed Grape Leaves *174*

*Square Meat Pies (*Sfeeha*)* *175*

Dumplings in Yogurt Sauce *176*

Stuffed Squash Casserole *177*

Beef and Potatoes with Tahini Sauce *178*

Stuffed Eggplant Casserole *179*

Lamb Chops *180*

Roast Leg of Lamb *181*

Lamb Meatballs *182*

Braised Lamb and Tomatoes *183*

Lamb and Rice Pockets *184*

15   Chicken Entrées **185**

Chicken Shawarma *186*

Spiced Chicken and Rice *187*

Chicken Roulade *188*

Roasted Chicken *189*

Mediterranean Meatloaf *190*

Chicken Kefta Kabob *191*

Chicken Skewers (Shish Tawook)..192

Chicken and Potatoes..193

Braised Chicken..194

Grilled Chicken on the Bone...195

16   Seafood Suppers 197

Fish and Rice (Sayadieh)..198

Spiced Fish..199

Pan-Seared Cod with Cherry Tomatoes......................................200

Salmon with Pesto..201

Baked Salmon...202

Tilapia with a Light Olive Sauce..203

17   Vegetarian Entrées.......................................205

Vegetarian Quinoa Pilaf...206

Vegetarian Bowtie Veggie Pasta..207

Vegetarian Couscous-Stuffed Tomatoes......................................208

Vegetarian Stuffed Baked Potatoes...209

Vegetarian Stuffed Squash..210

Vegetarian Baked Spaghetti..211

Vegetarian Potato Kibbeh...212

Vegetarian Cabbage Rolls...213

18   Sensational Side Dishes 215

Brown Rice with Vermicelli Noodles...216

Spicy Herb Potatoes (Batata Harra)...217

Green Fava Beans...218

Yellow Rice...219

Pickled Persian Cucumbers...220

Pickled Turnips (Kabees)...220

Dandelion Greens...221

Spiced Meat and Rice...222

Sautéed Zucchini and Mushrooms..223

Part 6:   Delectable Desserts.....................................225

19   Cookies, Baklava, and More 227

Pistachio Cookies..228

Date Cookies...229

Holiday Date Cookies (Maamoul)..230

Chocolate-Dipped Pistachio Sugar Cookies................................231

Jam Cookies...232

Baklava......233

Chocolate-Peanut Baklava......234

Date Balls......235

Fig Bars......236

Fig Puffs......237

Coconut Puffs (Macaroons)......238

20 Crave-Worthy Cakes......**239**

*Eggless Farina Cake (*Namoura*)*......240

*Turmeric Cake (*Sfoof*)*......241

Yogurt Cake......242

Date Cake......243

Olive Oil Cake......244

Yellow Cake with Jam Topping......245

Mediterranean Doughnuts......246

Mediterranean Cheesecakes......247

21 More Tempting Treats......**249**

*Halva (*Halawa*)*......250

Custard Cookie Trifle......251

Rice Pudding......252

*Mediterranean Bread Pudding (*Aish el Saraya*)*......253

*Shredded Phyllo and Sweet Cheese Pie (*Knafe*)*......254

Fried Pancakes......255

*Custard-Filled Pancakes (*Atayef*)*......256

*Phyllo Custard Pockets (*Shaabiyat*)*......257

Ashta Custard......258

*Sweet Cheese Rolls (*Halawet el Jibn*)*......259

Mascarpone-Stuffed Dates......260

Mediterranean Fruit Tart......261

Fruit Salad......262

Simple Syrup......263

*Turkish Coffee (*Greek Coffee*)*......264

Cinnamon Tea......265

Glossary......**267**

Index......**279**

Introduction

More and more people are discovering the numerous health benefits of the Mediterranean diet. If you're looking for a lifestyle change, or if you just want to feel better about what you eat, this book and this diet can help you get there.

In this book, you learn the basics of the Mediterranean diet and learn everything you need to know to get started on this health-promoting diet and lifestyle. I also help you discover a world of flavor and cooking you may have never tried before. And to help you get started on—and stick with—the diet, I also share more than 200 tastefully tantalizing breakfast, lunch, dinner, snack, and dessert recipes you and your family will love. Each recipe contains helpful nutritional information so you know how much of what you're putting into your body.

This isn't a diet plan on which you'll be miserable and eating bland, flavorless food. In fact, just the opposite is true. You'll enjoy fresh, natural foods just like the people who live along the borders of the Mediterranean Sea enjoy.

How This Book Is Organized

I've divided this book into six parts:

Part 1, What the Mediterranean Diet's All About, gives you background information on what exactly the Mediterranean diet is all about. I share why this diet is so healthy, explain the benefits of the ingredients, and give you tips on getting started on the diet.

In **Part 2, Mediterranean Breakfasts and Brunches,** I give you some healthy breakfast recipes to start off your day. These recipes are filled with complex carbohydrates, protein, and natural sugars from fruits—just what you need to jump-start your metabolism.

The recipes in **Part 3, Lunch on the Mediterranean,** are full of flavor and healthy ingredients. These dishes provide the right nutrition to give you the energy you need to fuel you through your day.

Snacks can be tricky when you're trying to lose weight or eat healthy because they can be filled with high amounts of calories. **Part 4, Snacks, Sauces, and More,** provides some healthy snacks that can give you the right kind of pick-me-up.

Main dishes can be very important because it could be the only meal you share with your family during the day. The main dish recipes in **Part 5, Mouthwatering Mediterranean Mains,** are filled with ingredients your family will enjoy while they reap the healthy benefits from all the nutrition.

The recipes in **Part 6, Delectable Desserts,** include many tasty ingredients like nuts, fruit, dates, and figs. These desserts are sweet and tasty, but as with all sweets, should be enjoyed in moderation.

At the back of the book, I've included a helpful glossary of terms to further your knowledge of the Mediterranean diet.

Extras

Throughout the book, you'll find bits of extra information to help you along your journey to a healthier way of eating:

DEFINITION

Turn to these sidebars for explanations of terms you might not know.

HEALTHY HINT

Healthy Hint sidebars offer tips on making healthier choices.

MEDITERRANEAN MORSEL

Check these sidebars for fun facts and interesting information about the Mediterranean diet.

TASTY TIP

These sidebars give you easy ideas on varying ingredients in a recipe for exciting new flavors.

Acknowledgments

This book is one of the most exciting projects I have worked on, and without Brook Farling, it would not be possible. Thanks Brook, for the opportunity to create this amazing book and to put my years of recipe testing on paper. I would also like to thank my followers and fans, without whom I would not have continued to work hard on creating recipes and educating people on the wonderful benefits of the Mediterranean diet. A special thank you to Mary Rodavich for lending her expertise and reviewing the recipes and providing the nutritional information. I know it was a lot of recipes, and you did an excellent job.

I want to dedicate this book to my amazing husband, Crisantos. You are the constant force pushing me to take that scary step forward. You are my partner and cheerleader, and without you, I would have never brought my love of cooking to the world. To my little angel and best friend, London, I love you with every beat of my heart, and you light up my life. To my amazing mom, Wafa, you are the master chef, I've learned everything about cooking from you, and you are the ever-present teacher telling me to add a little more salt. To my incredible dad, Hani, you are my role model, and you taught me how to live in this world and be the strongest and most amazing me that I could be. To my loving and always-supportive siblings, Angela, Haidar, and Nadeen, thank you for the endless encouragement to keep blazing ahead; you are my teammates for life. To my in-laws, Farid and Terry, thank you for the constant love and support. Thank you to my brother in-law, Joe, for always being in my corner. Kisses to my nieces, Amira, Athena, and Aaliyah, you are my rays of sunshine and I love you. To my best friend, Fatmi, we've been on this road for 25 years and there's still a ways to go. A big kiss and thank you to the rest of my wonderful family and friends.

Special Thanks to the Technical Reviewer

Idiot's Guides: The Mediterranean Diet Cookbook was reviewed by an expert who double-checked the accuracy of what you'll learn here, to help us ensure this book gives you everything you need to know about eating healthfully and nutritionally on the Mediterranean diet. Special thanks are extended to Mary Rodavich, MS, RD.

Trademarks

All terms mentioned in this book that are known to be or are suspected of being trademarks or service marks have been appropriately capitalized. Alpha Books and Penguin Group (USA) Inc. cannot attest to the accuracy of this information. Use of a term in this book should not be regarded as affecting the validity of any trademark or service mark.

What the Mediterranean Diet's All About

Welcome to the Mediterranean diet! In Part 1, I give you some key background information about the Mediterranean diet and explain all the benefits this diet—and lifestyle—offers. You learn how following this diet can help prevent a list of chronic diseases, discover the numerous nutritional benefits, and gain an understanding of how this diet helps you lose weight and maintain that weight loss.

You also learn how the diet works and how to get your family involved in—and excited about—all the changes. But change doesn't happen overnight, so I give you lots of advice and guidance on transitioning to this wonderful diet.

Armed with the knowledge in the chapters in Part 1, you set yourself up for success on the Mediterranean diet.

What Is the Mediterranean Diet?

What do you think of when someone says "Mediterranean food"? For me, fresh fruits and vegetables and flavorful herbs and spices come to mind. Mediterranean food encompasses these and all the other wonderful food and ingredients grown and prepared in the countries that border the Mediterranean Sea. These fresh and flavorful foods form the basis of the Mediterranean diet.

The Mediterranean diet is not just another diet fad. Rather, it's a whole way of life—a way of life millions of people residing along the Mediterranean Sea have been thriving on for thousands of years. A way of life that incorporates an array of flavorful and healthy ingredients such as olives, olive oil, bulgur wheat, figs, dates, grapes, tomatoes, legumes, chickpeas, and an array of tantalizing spices. A way of life you, too, can adopt.

In This Chapter

- Why the Mediterranean?
- The advantages of this way of eating
- The foods and flavors of the Mediterranean diet
- The benefits of exercise and stress reduction
- Dining out on the Mediterranean diet

A Little History

The Mediterranean diet was first brought to light by American scientist Dr. Ancel Keys. In the late 1950s, Keys conducted the Seven Countries Study, which followed the eating and lifestyle habits of participants in seven different countries—the United States, Finland, the Netherlands, Italy, the former Yugoslavia, Greece, and Japan.

Keys' findings showed that eating habits, type of fat consumption, and physical activity greatly decreased the study participants' risk of cardiovascular disease. What's more, it highlighted the fact that the people who had already embraced this diet and lifestyle lived along the Mediterranean Sea.

Since Keys' work, hundreds of other studies have been conducted and continue to support his findings of the many benefits of the Mediterranean diet.

The Benefits of the Mediterranean Diet

The health benefits of the Mediterranean diet are long lasting. Proven research has shown that following the Mediterranean diet prevents many chronic diseases. It also leads to an overall healthier lifestyle that includes physical and mental good health.

But the health benefits aren't attributed to diet alone. It's the combination of the nutritional portion with physical activity and relaxing leisure time that lead to the health benefits that have become so well documented.

Disease Prevention

Those who follow the Mediterranean diet have a decreased risk of cardiovascular disease, type 2 diabetes, cancer, Parkinson's disease, and Alzheimer's disease. But that's not all. Following the Mediterranean diet also improves brain function, reduces depression, and even prevents arthritis.

Cardiovascular disease is one of the largest contributors to death all over the world. A large portion of the Mediterranean diet comes from plant-based foods, including grains, legumes and nuts, and foods low in saturated fats. These, in turn, help lower abdominal obesity and reduce heart disease. Also, following a diet that's low in saturated fats and higher in fiber reduces cholesterol and high blood pressure.

Type 2 diabetes is a big problem, but it can be kept under control while adhering to the Mediterranean diet. Incorporating omega-3 fatty acids from fish, nuts, low-fat dairy products, and high-fiber foods helps control insulin levels and prevents the onset of diabetes. In addition, the lower occurrence of obesity and abdominal fat as a result of the Mediterranean diet reduces the chances of even developing type 2 diabetes.

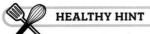 **HEALTHY HINT**

Consuming a Mediterranean-type diet rich in fruits, vegetables, and low-fat dairy products and reduced in sodium and saturated fat represents an ideal eating pattern. Weight loss and increased physical activity contribute to ideal lifestyle conditions.

—"The Evidence for Dietary Prevention and Treatment of Cardiovascular Disease," *Journal of the American Dietetics Association*

Eating foods high in omega-3 fatty acids, such as extra-virgin olive oil and nuts, can help keep your brain working properly—preventing or even slowing the onset of both Alzheimer's and Parkinson's diseases. The brain is made up of almost 60 percent fat, so eating healthy fats helps improve brain activity and increases the rate at which the brain repairs itself if it's injured or damaged by a stroke.

Research also shows that the Mediterranean diet lowers the risk of many types of cancer. Boosting your intake of extra-virgin olive oil, for example, contributes to a lower risk of breast cancer in women. The high amount of antioxidants and carotenoids found in plant-based foods, legumes, and whole grains also reduces the risk of other types of cancers and helps your body dispose of the free radicals that can cause this disease.

When it comes to depression, you are what you eat. If you're eating unhealthy amounts of saturated fats, processed food, and high amounts of sodium and sugar, that takes a toll on your body and your mental state. Your brain responds to what you put into your body, so if you're consuming unhealthy ingredients, eventually your digestive system, your organs, and your brain will be affected. In fact, the latter might become less responsive with less activity due to the inadequate nutrients it's receiving and absorbing.

In many of these instances, reducing your weight helps prevent several diseases, but improving the quality of ingredients you consume can help keep these diseases at bay as well.

Weight Loss

When you hear or see the word *diet,* do you picture bland, boring, flavorless food? Many people do. But with the Mediterranean diet, that's not the case at all. On the Mediterranean diet, you consume fresh, ripe, flavorful food—including fat. Some nutritionists view the Mediterranean diet as high in fat—and it is—but it's a *healthy* fat, mostly unsaturated, and from plant-based sources like olive oil.

The Mediterranean diet is not a quick fix. You won't see the pounds drop off immediately, but you will *feel* the difference. Adapting the Mediterranean diet is a lifestyle change, and with any lifestyle change, it takes time. You'll feel better overall as you adopt the changes to your eating habits because you'll be eating healthier foods. Adopting the Mediterranean diet will help you lose weight and sustain the weight loss over long periods of time.

 HEALTHY HINT

Omega-3 fatty acids found in fish oil may have the power to dramatically boost your metabolism—by about 400 calories per day, researchers from the University of Western Ontario report. Fish oil increases levels of fat-burning enzymes and decreases levels of fat-storage enzymes in your body. The great part of the Mediterranean diet is that you incorporate fish into your meal plan at least twice a week.

Making the transition to this healthier lifestyle requires a shift in thinking. You'll change how you shop for groceries, think differently about what you order off restaurant menus, and learn what recipes you like and what you want to incorporate into your meals. It also takes effort to work in physical activity into your day, but doing so helps your physical and mental health.

While making changes to what you eat, you'll also have to make changes to how you eat. Weight loss has a lot to do with calorie consumption. To lose weight, you have to create a calorie deficit, taking in less calories than you burn. It's easy to do this by exercising portion control—use smaller plates and then only eat what you put on your plate. Everyone has a different metabolic rate, which affects how fast you burn calories. Adding exercise to your day helps increase lean muscle, therefore, helping your metabolic rate.

Incorporating exercise and creating a calorie deficit is one part, but another part is what you eat. Eating foods higher in fiber and protein boosts your metabolism because they take more energy for your body to process, keeping you feeling full longer.

Superb Nutrition

One guarantee of the Mediterranean diet is the nutritional value of the foods you eat. The combination of nutritious foods you sample on this diet all work together to boost the amount of nutrients you take in. Antioxidants, carotenoids, fiber, protein, omega-3, vitamins, minerals, and unsaturated fats—none of these can be replaced by a supplement.

The maximum nutrition you get all depends on how much effort you put into the variety of foods you put on your plate. If you only practice certain parts of the Mediterranean diet and leave out others, you won't reap all the benefits that come with this lifestyle.

The key word here is *lifestyle*. This is more than a diet; it's a new way of thinking and living.

Components of the Mediterranean Diet and Lifestyle

Wouldn't it be nice if you could just pick up and move to one of the beautiful countries with a breathtaking diamond blue coastline along the Mediterranean Sea? Unfortunately, if you're like most people, that's not an option. You probably can't afford to hire a personal chef to organize and buy ingredients and prepare your meals, either. But doing it yourself isn't difficult.

Many people who live along the Mediterranean don't think of their eating habits as a diet—it's just their way of life. Eating fresh, plant-based ingredients and getting regular physical activity is how they've lived for thousands of years.

There's no subscription to prepackaged Mediterranean diet meals you can buy, and there really isn't a calorie meal plan you have to follow. You don't have to ban any one food group, and you don't have to avoid carbs. Instead, you'll be more conscious and mindful of how you eat every day—just like the millions of people along the Mediterranean Sea.

Not every single country along the Mediterranean eats the same way, but most do embrace many aspects of the Mediterranean diet as part of their culture and way of living. The type of food consumed differs based on country, culture, agriculture, and even regions within each country. In this book, I give you an overview of the diet and lifestyle.

Several key components combine to make this diet and lifestyle work:

- Eating fresh, in-season fruits and vegetables

- Reducing processed foods

- Using whole grains in everyday recipes

- Using "good" fats or unsaturated fats, from extra-virgin olive oil, nuts, fish, and avocados

- Eating moderate amounts of dairy in the form of cheese and Greek yogurt, which has lots of probiotics great for your digestive system

- Consuming lean protein from chicken, fish, eggs, and lean red meat in moderation

- Filling your diet with legumes, including beans, seeds, and nuts

- Using fresh and dried herbs and spices to boost flavor

- Drinking red wine, in moderation (This isn't necessary if you don't consume alcohol.)

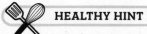

HEALTHY HINT

Red wine is a common part of Mediterranean meals, but imbibe in moderation to reap the benefits. Red wine contains health-promoting factors, including antioxidants, anti-inflammatories, and flavonoids. You can also get these benefits from drinking grape juice and eating dark berries if red wine isn't your forte.

- Getting daily exercise
- Reducing your stress level
- Making time for family, whether it's eating together or doing a fun activity

These are some basic things to remember, but what's most important is to incorporate each item in a way that suits you so you're more likely to continue to follow these tips.

On the Menu: Fresh, Nutritious Food

One of the most important parts of the Mediterranean diet is fresh—fresh fruits, fresh vegetables, fresh herbs, etc. You'll find very little processed food on this diet. What you will find is far more flavor and far fewer preservatives and sodium. Many of the dishes are brought to life by using herbs and spices instead of other, not-so-good-for-you ingredients.

This diet is thousands of years old, dating to a time when you couldn't find all types of fruits and vegetables available 365 days a year like you can today. People ate what was in season. This is a good practice because in-season fruits and vegetables actually have more nutrients than when they're out of season.

Buying local products also helps ensure you get the freshest ingredients. Fruits and vegetables lose nutrients the longer they sit in the refrigerator, so buying from local growers lets you know what you're getting is freshly picked and still contains many beneficial nutrients. But when fresh isn't available, people along the Mediterranean have learned to preserve food without using high amounts of salt, sugar, or fat by drying beans and grains and drying and pickling vegetables.

Another key to the Mediterranean diet is that although about 35 percent of your caloric intake comes from fat, it comes from *monounsaturated* fats—or healthy fats from olive oil, nuts, avocados, and fish. Nuts are a large part of the Mediterranean diet and contribute to your protein intake as well. Incorporating a handful of nuts every day can help boost your protein, omega-3 fatty acids, good fats, vitamin E, and fiber while reducing cholesterol.

Making Time for Exercise

In the Mediterranean culture, exercise is simply part of daily life. People do a lot of walking—and who wouldn't with the nice weather and stunning views around the Mediterranean Sea! Whether it's waking up early to take a stroll, walking to the grocery store, or sweeping the yard, physical activity isn't given a second thought.

But chances are, your scenery isn't as lovely to inspire you to get out and walk or do another form of exercise. In fact, maybe you dread exercise because the gym is too busy when you go, you're too tired before or after work, or you just have so much to do …. There's always an excuse—believe me, I've used them all!

It's up to you to decide what physical activity you enjoy, figure out how you can make it part of your life, and stick with it until it becomes habit. Many different forms of exercise are available that you can integrate into your daily life, such as walking during your lunch break, walking the kids to the park instead of driving, going for a bike ride on a Saturday morning instead of watching cartoons, walking between stores instead of driving when you're out shopping, or playing a sport the entire family can enjoy.

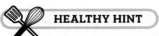 **HEALTHY HINT**

> If you have children, you can set an example that physical activity should be part of their lives as well.

Physical activity is an integral part of the Mediterranean diet, and in order to be successful when adopting the Mediterranean diet, you must integrate exercise into your life as well as making healthy eating choices.

Reducing Stress

As you're probably realizing by now, there's so much more to the Mediterranean diet and lifestyle than just food. It's also about making small changes to your daily life that improve the overall quality of your health—and that includes reducing your stress levels.

In many Mediterranean countries, taking a 2-hour break in the middle of the day to have lunch and take a nap is normal. But that's in the Mediterranean region. Maybe you can't take a 2-hour midday break, but you can definitely incorporate ways to reduce your stress throughout your day.

Try to get some sort of physical activity every day. It can be something as casual as walking your children to the park, or walking your dog for 20 minutes without looking at your phone and just enjoying nature. If you can't do something physical, try preparing a cup of coffee or tea, disconnecting from technology, and sitting on your porch to relax and sip it for 20 minutes. It's the little things that allow your body and mind to relax.

Family Time

Family is a big part of the Mediterranean culture. Family get-togethers aren't just during the holidays or special events in the Mediterranean culture. They're held every few days or at least once a week, creating a bond among everyone at the table.

In the fast-paced and highly technical era we live in, it's sometimes hard to make time for family. However, it should be a priority. Try planning dinner times so everyone can sit and eat a meal together. It helps build relationships and connections.

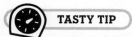 **TASTY TIP**

> Much research has shown that people with strong family interaction are less likely to suffer from depression.

If you don't have family nearby, you can create the same atmosphere with friends. Try planning weekly or bi-weekly get-togethers, and maybe have a different friend host it each time. Making meals potlucks takes the stress off any one person preparing a big meal. When you go, take a Mediterranean diet recipe to share with your friends!

Eating Out on the Diet

Sometimes eating out can be a problem no matter what diet plan or lifestyle you're following. Most items on restaurant menus are filled with salt, fat, and preservatives, making them off-limits.

But you can still dine out while on the Mediterranean diet. Find places to eat that align with your healthy eating habits, such as fresh fruit and vegetable items instead of fried or sauce-laden sides. Also choose menu items that aren't cooked in butter or heavy sauces, and ask for sauces or dressing to be served on the side, so you can control how much you consume.

Ask your server for recommendations, too, or see if he or she could ask the chef to make adjustments for you. You could request a lighter dressing, or ask for something to be grilled instead of fried. Remember, you're paying for it, so don't be afraid to politely ask for what you want.

Changing for the Better

Changing your eating habits to follow the Mediterranean diet can be very exciting. Knowing that you're making the conscious decision to improve your diet—and life—in a positive way and eat healthier is the first step of the Mediterranean diet.

It might seem overwhelming at first, but you don't have to make all the changes in one day. The more small changes you make, the more benefits you'll see, which will inspire you to make more beneficial changes. Those benefits will pay off big in the long run—for you and your family.

The Least You Need to Know

- The Mediterranean diet offers excellent disease prevention benefits.
- The Mediterranean diet is based on fresh, healthy ingredients bursting with flavor and nutrition.
- Getting exercise and reducing stress are key components of the Mediterranean lifestyle. Make them part of yours, too!
- Opt for foods that align with the Mediterranean diet when dining out, don't be afraid to ask about ingredients.
- The Mediterranean diet is more than a diet—it's a lifestyle. The more you change your thinking about it, the more benefits you can reap.

The Mediterranean Kitchen

Stocking your pantry is so important when adopting a new way of eating. You don't want to be stuck with a pantry empty of healthy foods and only chips or boxed cake mix as your meal or snack options. Keeping a well-stocked pantry gives you more alternatives and ideas of dishes you can make. Experimenting with different herbs, spices, and flavors is also important because these are low-calorie and fat-free ways of adding tremendous amount of flavor to any dish, all completely guilt free.

In this chapter, I give you the tools you need to begin this journey to a better way of eating—and a better way of life. The best place to start is by discovering what the Mediterranean diet food pyramid looks like. As you become familiar with the different categories and how many servings of each type of food you need to stay on track with the Mediterranean diet, you also discover what ingredients benefit you the most.

In This Chapter

- A look at the Mediterranean diet pyramid
- The main ingredients of the Mediterranean diet
- Herbs, spices, and other flavorings
- Stocking your kitchen and pantry

The Mediterranean Diet Pyramid

The Mediterranean kitchen is full of flavor and freshness. The dishes are brought to life with fresh herbs, dried herbs, and spices. Before you start cooking and eating, however, you need to understand the Mediterranean diet pyramid.

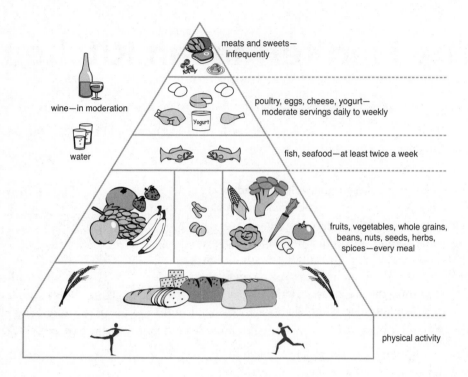

Oldways, the Harvard School of Public Health, and the European Office of the World Health Organization introduced the Mediterranean diet pyramid in 1993. The pyramid is based on the eating habits of inhabitants of the countries of Crete, Greece, and southern Italy in the 1960s. The pyramid has withstood the change in food trends from the past 50 years and remains the standard for eating to promote a longer and healthier lifestyle with less chronic disease.

In 2008, the Mediterranean diet pyramid received some minor updates. All plant foods—fruits, vegetables, grains, nuts, legumes, seeds, olives, and olive oil—are now grouped together and form the largest part of the pyramid. Also, herbs and spices are part of the current pyramid. They add flavor and aroma and reduce the need for fat and salt when cooking. Finally, fish and shellfish are recommended more often—at least twice a week—in recognition of their unique health benefits.

A large portion of the pyramid is dedicated to fruits, vegetables, grains, beans, nuts, legumes, herbs, spices, and olive oil. Physical activity and family time is another large part of the pyramid.

Here are some of the other key points of the pyramid:

- Choose fresh, less-processed fruits, vegetables, and grains to eliminate unneeded sodium and preservatives.
- Use olive oil (an unsaturated fat) for cooking, baking, and dressings.
- Eat cheese and Greek yogurt in moderation.
- Limit your intake of white sugar and salt.
- Eat more poultry and fish, and limit red meat to once a week.
- Drink water instead of sodas or sugary fruit drinks that could be filled with high-fructose corn syrup.

 MEDITERRANEAN MORSEL

You don't often see water in a food pyramid, but it's a very important part of any diet and lifestyle. About 60 percent of your body is composed of water, making it a very integral part of nutrition. Drinking water is an important habit to develop as you exercise. It also helps boost your metabolism.

Current food trends lean toward fast and easy. More and more people feel they're too busy to take the time to prepare a meal from scratch, and instead they resort to processed and ready-to-go meals. But all it takes is a little planning to provide your family with fresh, healthy, nutritious meals.

Mediterranean Foods and Ingredients

The quality of what you eat is as important as the ingredient itself. The Mediterranean diet contains many essential ingredients, and learning about each one helps you feel confident using it in recipes. Luckily, thanks to global trading, it's often easy to find these ingredients traditionally found only along the Mediterranean.

In the following sections, I introduce you to the ingredients you'll eat on the Mediterranean diet, highlight the importance of each ingredient, and tell you how to choose foods that suit your taste. Picking ingredients that conform to the Mediterranean diet is very important, but finding ones you actually like helps you enjoy and follow this way of life.

Fresh Fruits and Vegetables

Fruits and vegetables make up a large portion of the Mediterranean diet food pyramid, so let's look at them first. Fruits and vegetables are a very important part of any diet because they provide important vitamins, minerals, antioxidants, and fiber. Nutritionists suggest you consume five to nine servings of fruits and vegetables each day.

When purchasing fruits and vegetables, it's best to buy items that are in season, when they're at their peak flavor. (But if you really crave strawberries outside their season, that's okay, too.) Buying produce in season and as close to the time was picked ensures you get fruits or vegetables with the most nutrient. As fruits and vegetables sit, they lose nutrients. One way to ensure you're getting fresh produce is to buy from local farms and farmers' markets. When I purchase fruit or vegetables, I like to smell them. If the produce smells great, it's likely to taste great, too.

Let's look at fruits in particular. Fruits, regardless of where they're from, are good for you. They're full of flavor and nutrients; contain vitamins A, C, E; and are made mostly of water. What's more, they naturally contain little to no fat, cholesterol, or sodium.

Here are some key fruits on the Mediterranean diet:

Apples	Grapes
Apricots	Melons
Avocados	Olives
Bananas	Peaches
Berries	Pomegranate
Dates	Strawberries
Figs	

Fruits are easy to integrate into your daily diet plan. You can buy fruit that's easily transportable like apples, bananas, peaches, or apricots. Dried fruit is another great option. It's easy to pack and take with you, it won't spoil, it has intense flavor, and most of the nutrients are retained. Fruits are also great additions to your meals. Try adding dried fruit or pomegranate to salads, enhance the flavor of chicken with figs or dates, or add fresh fruit to a cup of Greek yogurt for a snack filled with protein and nutrients.

Fruits also contain natural sugars, which are easier for your body to digest and contain more nutrients than refined sugars. Natural sugars found in fruits are often called *fructose*. Although we've been trained to fear the word *sugar* and associate it with something bad, naturally occurring sugars are actually very important for the body.

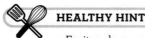 **HEALTHY HINT**

Fruit makes a great snack for the middle of the day. Instead of eating candy, chips, chocolate, or a cookie, reach for a piece of fruit you like. The sweet, refreshing taste will satisfy your sugar craving, and you won't end up with that sick feeling you get after eating too many cookies. What's more, you'll know you're doing something good for your body!

Now for vegetables. These good-for-you foods are another cornerstone of the Mediterranean diet. Vegetables are full of fiber, vitamins, minerals, chlorophyll, potassium, carotenoids, flavonoids, and antioxidants. They're also low in fat, sodium, and cholesterol. With the Mediterranean diet, vegetables should be the base of every meal and should take up half your plate.

So many different types of vegetables are popular on the Mediterranean diet. Here are a few to get you started:

Artichokes	Garlic
Beets	Leafy greens
Bell peppers	Onions
Carrots	Potatoes
Cauliflower	Romaine lettuce
Dandelion greens	Tomatoes
Eggplants	Zucchini

Vegetables are very nutritious and offer varying amounts and kinds of vitamins and minerals. They also give you a sizable amount of fiber, necessary for any diet. Vegetables are very low in calories, so eating a lot of vegetables can be very beneficial—they'll fill you up with good stuff!

 MEDITERRANEAN MORSEL

You might have noticed I put tomatoes on the vegetable list instead of with the fruit. Technically, tomatoes are a fruit, not a vegetable. But because most people recognize tomatoes as a veggie and prepare them like they do other vegetables, I put them in vegetables. Tomatoes and tomato products are a huge part of the Mediterranean diet, from fresh tomatoes, to tomato sauce, tomato paste, and so much more. They offer high amounts of antioxidants, vitamin C, and carotenoids, which is great for fighting and preventing cancer.

A large number of the recipes in this book, and from the Mediterranean region, include garlic and onions. These two ingredients can provide an abundance of flavor to any dish. They're versatile and can be cooked in different ways to alter their flavors and pungency, too. For example, when onions are sautéed slowly, they give off a sweet flavor, and when garlic is toasted in olive oil, it has a nutty flavor. Both also can be used raw atop a salad or in a dressing.

Also in the recipes, you'll see how often vegetables are easily integrated into the recipes and prepared in so many different ways. But remember that vegetables on their own are very healthy, so don't load them with heavy creams or sauces that add a lot of calories and fat. And keep in mind that the more vegetables you eat, the more your body benefits. So work them into your meal plan as often as you can.

Whole Grains

Whole grains are a large part of the Mediterranean diet. Full of fiber, vitamins, minerals, and complex carbohydrates, whole grains fill you up and help your digestive system. There are many types of whole grains—and as many ways to process them and foods made with them.

Here are some of the most common types of grains and whole grains used in the Mediterranean diet:

Barley	*Quinoa*
Brown rice	Spelt
Buckwheat	Whole rye
Bulgur	Whole-wheat flour
Corn	Whole-wheat pasta
Oats	

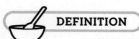

DEFINITION

Commonly thought of as a grain, **quinoa** is actually a nutty-flavored seed that's extremely high in protein and calcium.

Don't confuse refined grains with whole grains. Refined grains have been processed and the germ and bran layers have been removed. When the germ and bran layers are removed, much of the vitamins, minerals, and fiber are removed as well. What's left is mostly protein and starch.

The benefits of eating whole grains are numerous. They aid digestion; decrease cholesterol levels; assist with weight loss because they keep you full longer; and help prevent heart disease, stroke, cancer, and type 2 diabetes. Whole grains are very important to people who have diabetes because they help regulate blood insulin levels.

But not only are whole grains good for you; they taste great, too. Most of these grains have an earthy, nutty flavor. They're also easy to prepare in most cases.

Whole grains are extremely versatile. You can use them in soups; prepare them as pilafs; work them into breads, cakes, or cookies; or even use them as a stuffing. It's simple to make any dish a bit healthier by replacing all-purpose flour with whole-wheat flour, for example. Or replace long-grain rice with brown rice and regular pasta with whole-wheat pasta.

Legumes and Nuts

Legumes and nuts are another important part of the Mediterranean diet—in fact, they help make up the largest section of the diet, along with fruits, vegetables, and whole grains. Legumes are eaten green or harvested and dried for their beans or seeds, while nuts can be harvested from trees and plants.

Legumes include chickpeas, fava beans, lentils, peas, and white beans. These little seeds are full of nutrients, fiber, and protein. They also play an integral part in fighting and preventing chronic disease, and the soluble fiber they contain helps lower cholesterol, regulate insulin levels, assist digestion, and prevent cancer.

Legumes and their seeds are very inexpensive, and when dried, they last a long time. These ingredients are very popular in Mediterranean countries because they store easily and can be used throughout the winter, when traditionally the availability of meat or vegetables was low. Rehydrating them is very simple—just soak in water for a few hours and cook as desired. You can also rehydrate them, cook them in water, and freeze the cooked legumes. Then, when you're craving hummus, you can just defrost the beans in minutes, rather than a few hours. Using dried beans is also a great alternative to using canned goods, which can sometimes have numerous preservatives.

Nuts are common in the Mediterranean diet. They're tasty on their own or in many sweet or savory dishes. Whether roasted, toasted, or raw, walnuts, pine nuts, almonds, pistachios, sesame seeds, peanuts, cashews, and other nuts are full of flavor. The recipes later in the book demonstrate how easily you can add nuts to your diet.

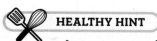 **HEALTHY HINT**

In a way, nuts are like vegetables: if you douse them with salt, sugar, and chocolate, you end up losing all of the benefits they offer. So skip the add-ons, and reap the benefits!

Unlike other foods in the Mediterranean diet pyramid's plant category, nuts actually contain fat—*unsaturated* fat. Therefore, nuts are considered heart healthy because they help lower bad cholesterol and prevent heart disease. They're also high in protein and are a great alternative to meat. Plus, nuts' fiber and antioxidants help your digestive system and slow cell aging.

However, nuts are high in calories, so eat in moderation. A handful a day can go a long way.

Meats, Poultry, and Eggs

The Mediterranean diet incorporates many different types of meats, including beef and lamb, poultry and eggs, and seafood, providing much-needed protein in small serving sizes. Meats are also a good source of iron. Animal products contain a type of iron called *heme iron,* which your body can absorb better than plant iron (called *nonheme iron*). Eating meat also helps in the absorption of plant iron.

Beef, lamb, and goat are common in the Mediterranean region. Along with sweets, you should limit your red meat intake. Once a week is enough, as long as you keep it within the recommended guidelines of only 12 to 16 ounces per month. Red meat is usually high in saturated fat, which is bad for your health and can cause heart disease, cholesterol, type 2 diabetes, and cancer.

When purchasing red meat, opt for the leanest cuts. Fillet, although it's very expensive, is a great cut of red meat because it's tender and very lean. You can grill it without adding any fat and can season it with fresh or dried herbs and spices to enhance the flavor. For ground meat, whether it's beef or lamb, I like to purchase a 95 percent lean, 5 percent fat ground. The small amount of fat helps keep the meat moist and flavorful. Adding spices can also boost the flavor.

Poultry and eggs are another great source of protein. Chicken, turkey, duck, and fowl are usually quite affordable and can be prepared in many different ways. To eliminate a lot of saturated fat when cooking poultry, remove the skin. And if you're looking for a leaner meat, use the breast. The recommended portion of poultry is 1 (6- to 8-ounce) serving every 2 days.

Over the years, eggs have received a bad reputation for being high in fat and cholesterol, but when you're on the Mediterranean diet, you should have no reason to avoid eggs. The Mediterranean diet actually *recommends* that you eat up to 7 eggs per week. Eggs are one of the best sources of high-quality protein and are still low in calories. They are rich in iron; folate; riboflavin; phosphorus; and vitamins A, D, and B_{12}. You can even find eggs that have omega-3s because the chickens who laid them were fed a certain diet.

Seafood is a great option for those who don't like poultry or red meat. It's high in protein, it's low in fat and calories, and it contains many different vitamins and minerals. Seafood also is a good source of omega-3 fatty acids, *EPA* (*eicosapentaenoic acid*) and *DHA* (*docosahexaenoic acid*).

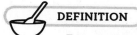 **DEFINITION**

Eicosapentaenoic acid (EPA) is a fatty acid that prevents blood clotting and helps reduce pain and swelling. It's used to regulate high blood pressure, heart disease, Alzheimer's disease, personality disorders, depression, and diabetes. **Docosahexaenoic acid (DHA)** is another fatty acid. It improves brain function, helps thin blood, and lowers triglyceride levels. It also reduces risk of type 2 diabetes, coronary artery disease, dementia, and attention deficit hyperactivity disorder.

When purchasing seafood, it's best to buy fresh fish from a good source—preferably a fishmonger who has a high volume of customers, so you know the fish hasn't been sitting in the display case more than 2 days. If the fish smells bad, it will taste bad, so don't buy it. And skip any cooked fish displayed next to raw fish to avoid cross-contamination. If you can't find fresh fish, your next best option is frozen. Just be sure to cook it immediately after defrosting it.

Stocking Your Pantry

Keeping your pantry stocked with fresh, healthy, nutritious foods helps ensure your success on the Mediterranean diet. Having such items on hand gives you more options when you're deciding what meals you want to make. And stocking up on the good stuff eliminates the temptation to reach for the bad stuff.

After reading through some recipes later in this book and deciding what you want to cook, you can easily put together a list of the foods and ingredients you'd like to have on hand. The following sections can help, too.

Spices and Herbs

Spices and herbs were added to the Mediterranean diet food pyramid in 2008 because they are such an essential component of the diet. Spices and herbs add an abundance of flavor without extra calories or fat. They also add some vitamins and minerals to your diet. And they're long-lasting: dried herbs and spices stay good for at least a year when stored in an airtight container.

Some recipes call for fresh herbs, while others call for dried. Why the difference? Flavor. The flavor of fresh herbs can be very earthy and pungent, while dried herbs are nuttier and toned down. You can add fresh herbs to recipes without needing to cook them, whereas dried herbs more than likely need to be cooked to bring out their flavor.

Here are some common herbs in the Mediterranean diet:

Basil	Oregano
Bay leaf	Parsley
Cilantro	Rosemary
Marjoram	Sage
Mint	Thyme

You can add a plethora of spices to Mediterranean diet recipes. Like herbs, spices add an abundance of flavor without any fat and calories. Spices also have nutritional benefits like lowering blood pressure and cholesterol.

Here are some common spices used in Mediterranean cooking:

Allspice	Cumin
Black pepper	Dried ginger
Cayenne	Paprika
Cinnamon	Sumac
Cloves	Zaatar
Coriander	

Salt

Salt enables you to get the most flavor from a dish. That's why you'll see salt called for in almost every recipe in this book—even desserts. Salt makes desserts taste sweeter because it awakens taste buds sensitive to salt and allows you to taste more.

The recipes in this book call for table salt because it's the most common type, but you can use sea salt instead if you like. It has more minerals and is an organic salt, while table salt is more processed.

Olive Oil

Olive oil, especially extra-virgin olive oil, is the main source of healthy fat in the Mediterranean diet. Its nutritional benefits are almost endless. Extra-virgin olive oil is an unsaturated fat; it contains polyphenols, antioxidants, and omega-3 fatty acids. These vitamins and minerals help lower cholesterol, reduce the risk of cancer, heart disease, arthritis, osteoporosis, and even type 2 diabetes.

There are different varieties of olive oil, each with its own flavor. *Extra-virgin olive oil* is the oil retrieved from the first press of the olives without any addition of heat. It usually has a stronger olive and fruity flavor and is also very low in acidity. *Virgin olive oil* is also made by pressing the olives without the addition of any heat, but the acidity levels are a bit higher and the flavor is a little less robust. Both *olive oil* and *light olive oil* are more refined and contain less nutrients and benefits than extra-virgin and virgin, and their flavors are much more subtle, making them great for baking as well.

All the varieties of olive oil have a low *smoking point*, which means they burn at a lower temperature than other oils.

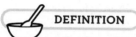 **DEFINITION**

Smoke point is the temperature at which an oil begins to break down or burn.

Picking a suitable olive oil for your taste buds makes your dishes more flavorful. Try incorporating the use of olive oil as your standard go-to fat in your kitchen.

Take care of your olive oil to make it last longer. Store extra-virgin olive oil in a dark glass bottle in a cool, dark place to keep the acidity levels low and the flavors intact.

Cheese and Yogurt

Although the recommended intake for dairy is only two servings per day, still opt for low-fat versions because dairy products are high in saturated fat. Avoid processed cheeses and instead choose fresh cheese made of sheep's or goat's milk. These are usually more flavorful, and a little goes a long way.

Greek yogurt, which has a thicker and creamier consistency than regular yogurt, is common in Mediterranean countries—and around the world. It contains live and active bacteria that aid your digestive and immune systems. Greek yogurt can be an ingredient or a side dish to many breakfast, lunch, or dinner recipes. It's readily available in most grocery stores, but if you want to make your own, I share a recipe in this book.

Honey, Waters, and Syrups

Honey is a natural sweetener that's superb for use in baked goods, desserts, breakfast, teas, and coffee. It contains 70 to 80 percent monosaccharides, fructose and glucose, which give it its sweet flavor. Research has shown that the antiseptic and antibacterial properties of honey can help with a cold or heal wounds.

Have you ever had orange blossom water or rose water? Neither has a huge nutritional value, but they both have intense flavors and add an exotic flavor element to any dessert or drink. You can find them at specialty food stores. They're fairly inexpensive.

Syrups in Mediterranean cooking are most commonly used for desserts, as a topping. Simple syrup, for example, is made from simmering sugar, water, a bit of lemon juice, and a flavoring such as orange blossom water or rose water. Then you can drizzle it on phyllo pastries, fruit, or yogurt to sweeten.

 MEDITERRANEAN MORSEL

Many apps and tools are available for smartphones and notepads to help you get organized. I like an app called Grocery iQ. It enables you to organize your grocery lists, create lists by store, keep a history of previous list items, and even sends you coupons.

The Least You Need to Know

- The Mediterranean diet pyramid serves as a good guide of what foods, and how much of them, you eat on the diet.
- Stocking your pantry and refrigerator with good-for-you Mediterranean-inspired ingredients means you're prepared to get creative with mealtimes.
- Olive oil is a key ingredient in the Mediterranean diet, and many are available. Find the versions you like best.
- Greek yogurt contains live probiotics that are great for your digestive and immune systems.

Mediterranean Breakfasts and Brunches

Part 2 is where the mouthwatering Mediterranean recipes start. In the following chapters, I share several recipes to get you started on a good start to your day.

From quick grab-and-go breakfasts for weekday mornings when you don't have time to sit and enjoy a leisurely meal to those weekend mornings when brunch is just what the day calls for, you'll find a variety of breakfast recipes—sweet as well as savory—worth waking up for.

Quick Breakfasts

Breakfast is the most important meal of the day. You've probably heard that saying numerous times, but for a reason—because it's true! The Mediterranean diet breakfast recipes in this chapter are hearty meals with complex carbohydrates and proteins that give you energy and fuel you through lunchtime.

A dominant ingredient in the breakfast of the Mediterranean diet is eggs, prepared many ways—fried, scrambled, hard-boiled, and in other tasty preparations, often combined with a protein or a vegetable. Eggs are readily available in Mediterranean countries. I remember visiting my grandmother's house in Lebanon and being awakened every morning by the roosters' crowing.

Another great part of the Mediterranean diet is being able to enjoy something sweet in the morning—yogurt, fruit, honey, or other natural unrefined sugars. Having something sweet in the morning has actually been shown to help people lose weight because it curbs cravings throughout the day.

In This Chapter

- Quick-and-easy weekday breakfasts
- Excellent eggs
- Hearty potato breakfasts

Yogurt Spread (*Labne*)

Labne is very popular as a breakfast food. It has a smooth, tangy flavor, and when you add garlic and mint to it, the flavor is enhanced even more. It's great to spread on toast, a bagel, or even pita.

Yield:	Prep time:	Serving size:	
1 1/2 cups	2 days	2 tablespoons	
Each serving has:			
23 calories	0g fat	0g saturated fat	4g protein
1g carbohydrate	0g dietary fiber	2mg cholesterol	14mg sodium

2 cups plain Greek yogurt   1 tsp. dried mint (optional)

1 tsp. minced garlic (optional)

1. Place a strainer over a bowl. Line the strainer with 2 layers of cheesecloth.

2. Pour Greek yogurt into the cheesecloth. Gently bring together the ends of the cheesecloth, and twist it to hold in yogurt. This helps liquid drain out.

3. Set the cheesecloth back in the strainer, and refrigerate for 2 days to drain.

4. Remove labne spread from the cheesecloth.

5. Stir in garlic (if using) and mint (if using), and store in a sealed container in the refrigerator.

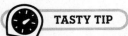 **TASTY TIP**

If you don't like garlic or mint, you don't have to use them in this recipe. The labne is just as good on its own as a spread.

Yogurt Bowl

This breakfast brings together some of the most important parts of the Mediterranean diet—tangy yogurt, fresh fruit, and sweet natural honey. It's full of protein and fiber.

Yield:	Prep time:	Serving size:	
2 cups	5 minutes	2 cups	
Each serving has:			
364 calories	1g fat	0g saturated fat	24g protein
64g carbohydrate	3g dietary fiber	12mg cholesterol	84mg sodium

1 cup plain Greek yogurt

$^1/_2$ medium banana, peeled and sliced

3 medium fresh strawberries, cored and sliced

$^1/_4$ cup fresh blueberries

2 TB. raw honey

1. Place Greek yogurt in a bowl. Top with banana slices, strawberry slices, and blueberries.

2. Drizzle honey over fruit, and serve cold.

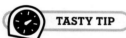 **TASTY TIP**

You can replace any of the fruit in this recipe with your favorites. If you can't have honey, try using maple syrup or 1 tablespoon of your favorite jam.

Quick Cream of Wheat

My grandmother used to make this breakfast for me whenever I'd sleep over. It's a warm, smooth, and creamy bowl of goodness.

Yield:	Prep time:	Cook time:	Serving size:
4 cups	5 minutes	12 minutes	1 cup

Each serving has:			
307 calories	21g fat	10g saturated fat	9g protein
22g carbohydrate	0g dietary fiber	47mg cholesterol	462mg sodium

4 cups whole milk	3 TB. sugar
1/2 cup *farina*	3 TB. butter
1/2 tsp. salt	3 TB. pine nuts

1. In a large saucepan over medium heat, bring whole milk to a simmer, and cook for about 4 minutes. Do not allow milk to scorch.

2. Whisk in farina, salt, and sugar, and bring to a slight boil. Cook for 2 minutes, reduce heat to low, and cook for 3 more minutes. Stay close to the pan to ensure it doesn't boil over.

3. Pour mixture into 4 bowls, and let cool for 5 minutes.

4. Meanwhile, in a small pan over low heat, cook butter and pine nuts for about 3 minutes or until pine nuts are lightly toasted.

5. Evenly spoon butter and pine nuts over each bowl, and serve warm.

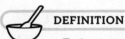 **DEFINITION**

Farina is a cereal grain often referred to as cream of wheat. It's usually served warm as a breakfast food but has many other uses in baking or pasta-making.

Garlic Scrambled Eggs

In this quick and easy breakfast, eggs are flavored with browned beef and toasted bits of garlic. The flavor gets up and going in the morning.

Yield:	Prep time:	Cook time:	Serving size:
2 cups	5 minutes	10 minutes	$^1/_2$ cup

Each serving has:			
188 calories	15g fat	4g saturated fat	11g protein
1g carbohydrate	0g dietary fiber	228mg cholesterol	378mg sodium

$^1/_4$ lb. ground beef	1 TB. garlic, finely chopped
2 TB. extra-virgin olive oil	4 large eggs
$^1/_2$ tsp. salt	$^1/_2$ tsp. ground black pepper

1. In a nonstick pan over medium heat, brown beef for 5 minutes, breaking up chunks with a wooden spoon.

2. Add extra-virgin olive oil, salt, and garlic, cook for 3 more minutes.

3. Break eggs into the pan, stir eggs into beef and garlic mixture, and cook for 2 more minutes.

4. Season with black pepper, and serve warm.

Holiday Eggs

My mom would make this egg dish for every holiday. It's a medley of flavorful ingredients: browned ground beef, sautéed onions and garlic, cut with sweet and tangy tomato sauce, and finished with creamy eggs.

Yield:	Prep time:	Cook time:	Serving size:
6 cups	5 minutes	20 minutes	1 cup

Each serving has:			
211 calories	16g fat	4g saturated fat	13g protein
3g carbohydrate	1g dietary fiber	234mg cholesterol	139mg sodium

$^1/_2$ lb. ground beef

$^1/_2$ medium yellow onion, chopped

1 tsp. minced garlic

$^1/_2$ tsp. salt

3 TB. extra-virgin olive oil

1 (15-oz.) can crushed tomatoes, with juice

6 large eggs

$^1/_2$ tsp. ground black pepper

1. In a medium skillet over medium heat, brown beef for 3 minutes, breaking up chunks with a wooden spoon.

2. Add yellow onion, garlic, salt, and extra-virgin olive oil, and cook for 5 minutes.

3. Pour in crushed tomatoes with juice, stir, and cook for 5 more minutes.

4. Add eggs to the skillet, stir into scramble, and cook for 3 more minutes.

5. Add black pepper, and serve warm.

Mediterranean Omelet

The options for omelet ingredients are nearly limitless. This version boasts a medley of fresh Mediterranean flavors.

Yield:	Prep time:	Cook time:	Serving size:
1 omelet	5 minutes	10 minutes	1 omelet

Each serving has:			
560 calories	49g fat	12g saturated fat	20g protein
13g carbohydrate	6g dietary fiber	450mg cholesterol	1,891mg sodium

2 TB. extra-virgin olive oil

2 TB. yellow onion, finely chopped

1 small clove garlic, minced

$^1/_2$ tsp. salt

1 cup fresh spinach, chopped

$^1/_2$ medium tomato, diced

2 large eggs

2 TB. whole or 2 percent milk

4 kalamata olives, pitted and chopped

$^1/_2$ tsp. ground black pepper

3 TB. crumbled feta cheese

1 TB. fresh parsley, finely chopped

1. In a nonstick pan over medium heat, cook extra-virgin olive oil, yellow onion, and garlic for 3 minutes.

2. Add salt, spinach, and tomato, and cook for 4 minutes.

3. In a small bowl, whisk together eggs and whole milk.

4. Add kalamata olives and black pepper to the pan, and pour in eggs over sautéed vegetables.

5. Using a rubber spatula, slowly push down edges of eggs, letting raw egg form a new layer, and continue for about 2 minutes or until eggs are cooked.

6. Fold omelet in half, and slide onto a plate. Top with feta cheese and fresh parsley, and serve warm.

Potatoes and Eggs Omelet

This isn't your typical potatoes-and-eggs dish. Seasoned potatoes, ground beef, and spices are cooked into an omelet. It's all you need to start the day.

Yield:	Prep time:	Cook time:	Serving size:
1 omelet	10 minutes	14 minutes	$^1/_4$ omelet

Each serving has:			
249 calories	15g fat	4g saturated fat	13g protein
15g carbohydrate	2g dietary fiber	228mg cholesterol	384mg sodium

$^1/_4$ lb. ground beef

1 large potato, washed and grated

2 TB. extra-virgin olive oil

$^1/_2$ tsp. salt

$^1/_2$ tsp. *seven spices*

4 large eggs

$^1/_2$ tsp. ground black pepper

1. In a nonstick pan over medium heat, brown beef for 5 minutes, breaking up chunks with a wooden spoon.

2. Add grated potato, extra-virgin olive oil, salt, and seven spices, and cook for 7 minutes or until potatoes are lightly browned.

3. Break eggs into a bowl, and whisk together.

4. Gently pour eggs into meat and potato mixture.

5. Using a rubber spatula, slowly push down edges of eggs, letting raw egg form a new layer, and continue for about 2 minutes or until eggs are cooked.

6. Season with black pepper, and serve warm.

 DEFINITION

Seven spices is a spice mix used to season many Mediterranean dishes. I share my go-to recipe in Chapter 13.

Herbed Potatoes and Eggs

Potatoes and eggs go hand in hand for almost any breakfast dish, but it's not very often you see these ingredients prepared this way. The smooth texture and flavor of the boiled eggs and potatoes are livened by fresh herbs.

Yield:	Prep time:	Cook time:	Serving size:
6 cups	30 minutes	32 minutes	1 cup
Each serving has:			
136 calories	3g fat	1g saturated fat	6g protein
21g carbohydrate	2g dietary fiber	141mg cholesterol	441mg sodium

2 large potatoes

4 large eggs, at room temperature

1 tsp. salt

$^{1}/_{2}$ tsp. ground black pepper

2 TB. fresh parsley, chopped

2 whole green onions, finely chopped

1. In a large saucepan, add potatoes along with enough water to cover potatoes by 1 inch. Set over medium heat, bring to a simmer, and cook for 25 minutes.

2. Pour off water, and set potatoes aside to slightly cool.

3. Add eggs to a medium saucepan, pour in enough water to cover eggs, and set over medium heat. Bring to a boil, cook for 2 minutes, and remove from heat. Cover, and set aside for 15 minutes.

4. Remove eggs, place in a bowl of cold water, and let sit for 10 minutes.

5. Peel potatoes and eggs, and place in a large bowl. Season with salt and black pepper, and mash using a potato masher for about 1 minute or until the texture resembles medium chunks.

6. Add parsley and green onions, and toss well.

7. Serve warm with pita bread and Greek yogurt.

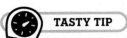 **TASTY TIP**

If you don't like parsley or green onions, you can use fresh thyme or chives instead.

Fried Cheese

This fried cheese is often served for breakfast and sometimes even as an appetizer. Halloumi has a great brine flavor with texture that holds up to frying.

Yield:	Prep time:	Cook time:	Serving size:
4 slices	10 minutes	8 minutes	1 slice

Each serving has:			
178 calories	14g fat	8g saturated fat	10g protein
4g carbohydrate	1g dietary fiber	29mg cholesterol	423mg sodium

6 oz. *halloumi cheese*	1 medium tomato, sliced
1 TB. extra-virgin olive oil	10 fresh mint leaves
1 medium Persian cucumber, sliced	

1. Slice halloumi cheese into 4 equal slices. Layer 2 paper towels, lay out cheese on the paper towels, let it dry for 3 minutes. Turn over cheese, and let dry for 3 more minutes.

2. Preheat a nonstick pan over medium-low heat. Add extra-virgin olive oil and cheese slices, and cook for 4 minutes per side or until golden brown.

3. Arrange cheese on a plate with sliced Persian cucumber, sliced tomato, and fresh mint leaves. Enjoy with pita bread.

 DEFINITION

Halloumi cheese is an unripened brined cheese that originated in Cyprus and is very popular in Greece, Turkey, and Lebanon. It has a high melting point, so it's great for frying or grilling.

Brunch Bites

Brunch is a leisurely meal, and the recipes in this chapter are great for weekend brunches. They take a little longer to prepare, but they're well worth the time.

Brunch doesn't have to be eggs and hashbrowns, pancakes, or waffles. Try new recipes that have a new array of tastes and ingredients. The brunch recipes in this chapter are full of flavor you'll love.

In This Chapter

- Delicious brunch dishes
- Weekend-worthy breakfasts
- Exploring new flavors

Breakfast Casserole (*Fatteh*)

My mom used to reserve this hearty breakfast casserole especially for the weekend. It's a layered casserole that includes crispy pita bread, hearty chickpeas, mini-meatballs, and a garlic-enhanced yogurt sauce.

Yield:	Prep time:	Cook time:	Serving size:
8 cups	30 minutes	30 minutes	1 cup

Each serving has:			
491 calories	34g fat	10g saturated fat	23g protein
26g carbohydrate	5g dietary fiber	56mg cholesterol	931mg sodium

1 (16-oz.) can chickpeas, rinsed and drained

$1^1/_2$ cups water

1 lb. ground beef

$1^1/_2$ tsp. salt

$^1/_2$ tsp. ground black pepper

2 cups Greek yogurt

2 TB. minced garlic

$^1/_2$ cup tahini paste

$^1/_4$ cup fresh lemon juice

$^1/_3$ cup butter

$^1/_2$ cup pine nuts

4 cups plain pita chips

$^1/_2$ cup fresh parsley, finely chopped

1. In a small saucepan over low heat, combine chickpeas and $^1/_2$ cup water. Simmer for 5 minutes, and remove from heat.

2. In a small bowl, combine beef, 1 teaspoon salt, and black pepper. Form mixture into about 20 to 30 mini meatballs about 1 teaspoon each.

3. Preheat a skillet over low heat. Add meatballs, cover, and cook for 5 minutes. Uncover, cook for 3 more minutes, and remove from heat.

4. In a medium bowl, whisk together Greek yogurt, garlic, tahini paste, lemon juice, remaining 1 cup water, and remaining $^1/_2$ teaspoon salt. Set aside.

5. In a separate small saucepan over low heat, melt butter. Add pine nuts, and toast for about 3 minutes or until lightly browned. Remove from heat.

6. In a large, 3-inch-deep casserole dish, evenly distribute pita chips. Layer chickpeas over top, and add a layer of mini-meatballs. Pour yogurt sauce over meatballs, sprinkle with pine nuts, and pour browned butter over top. Sprinkle with parsley, and serve warm.

MEDITERRANEAN MORSEL

If you don't have pita chips but you do have pita bread, you can make your own chips. Preheat your oven to 400°F, lay pita bread directly on the oven rack, and toast for 4 or 5 minutes. Be sure to keep your eye on the pita to be sure it doesn't burn. You want it to be brown but not burned. When it's toasted, just break it up with your hands.

Mediterranean Breakfast Quiche

This quiche brings together many Mediterranean flavors—basil, sun-dried tomatoes, parsley, onions, and garlic—to make a medley of bright flavors.

Yield:	Prep time:	Cook time:	Serving size:
8- or 9-inch quiche	45 minutes	1 hour	$1/8$ quiche

Each serving has:			
419 calories	23g fat	13g saturated fat	13g protein
27g carbohydrate	2g dietary fiber	158mg cholesterol	830mg sodium

$1^1/_2$ cups all-purpose flour	2 cups spinach, chopped
1 tsp. dried oregano	4 large eggs
$^1/_2$ tsp. garlic powder	$^1/_2$ cup heavy cream
2 tsp. salt	1 cup ricotta cheese
5 TB. cold butter	$^1/_3$ cup grated Parmesan cheese
3 TB. vegetable shortening	1 tsp. paprika
$^1/_4$ cup ice water	$^1/_2$ tsp. cayenne
3 TB. extra-virgin olive oil	$^1/_2$ tsp. ground black pepper
1 medium yellow onion, chopped	$^1/_4$ cup fresh basil, chopped
1 TB. minced garlic	$^1/_4$ cup fresh parsley, chopped
4 stalks asparagus, chopped	$^1/_3$ cup sun-dried tomatoes, chopped

1. In a food processor fitted with a chopping blade, pulse together $1^1/_2$ cups all-purpose flour, oregano, garlic powder, and $^1/_2$ teaspoon salt five times.

2. Add cold butter and vegetable shortening, and pulse for 1 minute or until mixture resembles coarse meal.

3. Continue to pulse while adding ice water, about 1 minute. Test dough—if it holds together when you pinch it, it doesn't need any more water. If it doesn't come together, add 3 more tablespoons cold water.

4. Remove dough from the food processor, put into a plastic bag, and form into a flat disc. Refrigerate for 30 minutes.

5. Preheat the oven to 400°F. Flour a rolling pin and your counter.

6. Roll out dough to $^1/_4$ inch thickness. Fit dough into an 8- or 9-inch tart pan. Using a fork, slightly puncture bottom of piecrust. Bake for 15 minutes. Remove from the oven, and set aside.

7. In a large skillet over medium heat, add extra-virgin olive oil, yellow onion, garlic, and asparagus, and sauté for 5 minutes.

8. Add spinach, and cook for 3 or 4 more minutes. Remove from heat, and set aside.

9. In a large bowl, whisk together eggs, heavy cream, and ricotta cheese. Add remaining $1^1/_2$ teaspoons salt, Parmesan cheese, paprika, cayenne, black pepper, basil, parsley, and sun-dried tomatoes, and stir to combine.

10. Pour filling into piecrust, and bake for 40 minutes. Remove from the oven, and let rest for 20 minutes before serving warm.

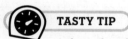 **TASTY TIP**

If you don't like spinach or asparagus, try adding a vegetable you do like. Broccoli, squash, or peppers all work well in this quiche.

Shanklish Cheese

This cheese is pungent and covered in earthy, dried herbs. In addition to a nice brunch dish, shanklish cheese is great over a salad or simply sliced with olive oil—either way the flavor is intense.

Yield:	Prep time:	Cook time:	Serving size:
3 cheese balls	3 days	15 minutes	1 cheese ball
Each serving has:			
396 calories	12g fat	2g saturated fat	47g protein
27g carbohydrate	5g dietary fiber	24mg cholesterol	560mg sodium

6 cups Greek yogurt

$^1/_2$ tsp. salt

$^1/_2$ tsp. cayenne

$^1/_2$ cup dried thyme

1 medium tomato, finely diced

$^1/_2$ medium yellow onion, finely chopped

2 TB. extra-virgin olive oil

1. In a large saucepan over low heat, bring Greek yogurt to a light boil. You'll see yogurt begin to curdle, and curd and whey will separate.

2. Lay two pieces of cheesecloth over a strainer, pour yogurt into the cheesecloth, and pour off excess moisture. Bring together the ends of the cheesecloth, and place the strainer over a bowl. Refrigerate for 2 days.

3. Remove cheese from the cheesecloth, and transfer to a bowl. Add salt and cayenne, and stir to combine.

4. Lay a double layer of paper towels on a plate. Form cheese into 2-inch balls, roll balls in thyme to cover completely, and place cheese on the paper towels. Cover with another layer of paper towels, and refrigerate for 24 hours to dry.

5. Store cheese in olive oil, or wrap in a paper towel and refrigerate for up to 2 weeks. When ready to serve, crumble cheese on a plate with tomatoes and yellow onion and drizzled with extra-virgin olive oil.

Cheesy Breakfast Pizza (*Cheese Manakish*)

Adults and children of all ages love this brunch pizza. Gooey melted cheese with soft, chewy bread—what's not to love?

Yield:	Prep time:	Cook time:	Serving size:
6 pizzas	20 minutes	10 minutes	1 pizza
Each serving has:			
699 calories	35g fat	14g saturated fat	36g protein
61g carbohydrate	3g dietary fiber	69mg cholesterol	1,169mg sodium

1 batch Multipurpose Dough (recipe in Chapter 12)

¼ cup all-purpose flour

2 cups *kashkaval cheese*, grated

2 cups mozzarella cheese, grated

1. Preheat the oven to 400°F. Flour a rolling pin and your counter.

2. Divide Multipurpose Dough into 6 equal portions, and roll out dough into 6- to 8-inch-diameter circles.

3. In a medium bowl, combine kashkaval cheese and mozzarella cheese. Divide cheese mixture into 6 portions, and sprinkle on each dough circle.

4. Place pizzas onto a baking sheet, and bake for 8 to 10 minutes or until cheese begins to bubble.

5. Remove pizzas from the oven, fold each pizza in half, and enjoy as is or with Yogurt Spread (Labne; recipe in Chapter 3).

 DEFINITION

Kashkaval cheese is a semihard yellow Bulgarian cheese that has a very bold flavor. Kashkaval comes in two types. One is made with cow's milk, and one is made with sheep's milk. If you like a more pungent flavor, use the sheep's milk version.

Thyme Breakfast Pizza (*Zaatar Manakish*)

This is a very traditional breakfast pizza. The tangy, earthy flavor of the zaatar seasoning along with the soft, chewy bread definitely wakes you up!

Yield:	Prep time:	Cook time:	Serving size:
6 pizzas	20 minutes	10 minutes	1 pizza
Each serving has:			
558 calories	30g fat	4g saturated fat	10g protein
64g carbohydrate	6g dietary fiber	0mg cholesterol	784mg sodium

1 cup zaatar $^1/_4$ cup all-purpose flour

$^1/_2$ cup extra-virgin olive oil

1 batch Multipurpose Dough
   (recipe in Chapter 12)

1. Preheat the oven to 400°F. Flour a rolling pin and your counter.

2. Divide Multipurpose Dough into 6 equal portions, and roll out dough into 6- to 8-inch-diameter circles.

3. In a small bowl, combine zaatar with extra-virgin olive oil. Spread 2 or 3 tablespoons zaatar mixture onto each dough circle.

4. Place pizzas onto a baking sheet, and bake for 8 to 10 minutes or until zaatar begins to bubble.

5. Remove pizzas from the oven, fold each pizza in half, enjoy as is or with Yogurt Spread (Labne; recipe in Chapter 3).

Breakfast Beans (*Ful Mudammas*)

Ful mudammas is a combination of chickpeas and fava beans mixed with a bright citrus dressing. This breakfast dish is full of protein, fiber, and flavor.

Yield:	Prep time:	Cook time:	Serving size:
3 cups	15 minutes	10 minutes	1 cup

Each serving has:			
336 calories	19g fat	3g saturated fat	9g protein
35g carbohydrate	8g dietary fiber	0mg cholesterol	1,374mg sodium

1 (15-oz.) can chickpeas, rinsed and drained	¹/₂ cup fresh lemon juice
1 (15-oz.) can fava beans, rinsed and drained	¹/₂ tsp. cayenne
1 cup water	¹/₂ cup fresh parsley, chopped
1 TB. minced garlic	1 large tomato, diced
1 tsp. salt	3 medium radishes, sliced
	¹/₄ cup extra-virgin olive oil

1. In a 2-quart pot over medium-low heat, combine chickpeas, fava beans, and water. Simmer for 10 minutes.

2. Pour bean mixture into a large bowl, and add garlic, salt, and lemon juice. Stir and smash half of beans with the back of a wooden spoon.

3. Sprinkle cayenne over beans, and evenly distribute parsley, tomatoes, and radishes over top. Drizzle with extra-virgin olive oil, and serve warm or at room temperature.

 MEDITERRANEAN MORSEL

This bean dish is loaded with fiber and protein. It'll energize you straight through to lunchtime.

Chicken Liver

Chicken liver can be a heavy meat to eat, but this recipe lightens it with citrus, garlic, and a refreshing push herbs.

Yield:	Prep time:	Cook	Serving size:
4^1/$_2$ cups	15 minutes	7 minutes	^{3}/$_4$ cup

Each serving has:			
246 calories	14g fat	3g saturated fat	26g protein
4g carbohydrate	0g dietary fiber	571mg cholesterol	483mg sodium

2 lb. chicken liver	^{1}/$_2$ tsp. ground black pepper
3 TB. extra-virgin olive oil	1 cup fresh cilantro, finely chopped
3 TB. minced garlic	^{1}/$_4$ cup fresh lemon juice
1 tsp. salt	

1. Cut chicken livers in half, rinse well, and pat dry with paper towels.

2. Preheat a large skillet over medium heat. Add extra-virgin olive oil and garlic, and cook for 2 minutes.

3. Add chicken liver and salt, and cook, tossing gently, for 5 minutes. Remove the skillet from heat, and spoon liver onto a plate.

4. Add black pepper, cilantro, and lemon juice. Lightly toss, and serve warm.

Sweet Bread with Dates

Tea is a big part of the Mediterranean diet, and if you're drinking tea for brunch, you need something to dunk into it! This sweet bread filled with a smooth sweet date paste is the perfect breakfast if you wake up with a sweet tooth.

Yield:	Prep time:	Cook time:	Serving size:
12 rolls	1 day plus 3 hours	30 minutes	1 roll

Each serving has:			
305 calories	11g fat	7g saturated fat	7g protein
46g carbohydrate	3g dietary fiber	80mg cholesterol	347mg sodium

2³/₄ cups all-purpose flour	¹/₃ cup plus 1 TB. water
¹/₄ cup dry milk	10 TB. butter
¹/₄ cup sugar	12 medjool dates, pitted
1¹/₄ tsp. salt	1 TB. orange blossom water
1 TB. instant yeast	¹/₂ tsp. cinnamon
3 large eggs	1 large egg white

1. In a food processor fitted with a dough attachment or in a blender, knead all-purpose flour, dry milk, sugar, salt, instant yeast, eggs, ¹/₃ cup water, and 8 tablespoons butter for 15 minutes.

2. Transfer dough to a bowl lightly sprayed with olive oil spray, cover the bowl with plastic wrap, and let rise in the refrigerator for 24 hours.

3. In a food processor fitted with a chopping blade, blend medjool dates, orange blossom water, and cinnamon for 2 minutes or until smooth.

4. Grease a 12-cup muffin tin with remaining 2 tablespoons butter.

5. Form dough into 12 equal pieces. Spoon 1 tablespoon date mixture into center of each dough piece, tightly seal dough around date mixture, and place seal side down into the prepared muffin tin.

6. Set aside dough to rise for 1 hour.

7. Preheat the oven to 375°F.

8. In a small bowl, whisk together egg white and remaining 1 tablespoon water. Brush each roll with egg wash.

9. Bake for 30 minutes.

10. Remove rolls from the oven, and let rest for 20 minutes before serving.

 MEDITERRANEAN MORSEL

If you're not familiar with orange blossom water, you're missing out! It has a light, flowery flavor with hints of citrus, and it adds a sweet and unique flavor to desserts and pastries.

Lunch on the Mediterranean

In the Mediterranean culture, lunch is a very important meal. People take lunch as a major break during the day and often even take a nap after lunch. And the lunch hour isn't just 30 minutes to an hour; more often it's closer to 2 hours, allowing people to go home, eat a filling meal, and relax so they're revived and renewed when they go back to work.

Coming in the middle of the day, lunch gives you the opportunity to give your body a much-needed energy boost. What's more, Mediterranean lunches often are as filling as the dinner meal, so you're sure to power through to dinner.

In Part 3, I give you flavorful Mediterranean recipes that wake up your taste buds. And talk about variety—salads, soups and stews, rice and grain dishes, and so much more—the chapters in Part 3 are sure to offer something you'll love for lunch.

Lovely Lunch Salads

Mediterranean salads highlight the fresh, healthy ingredients found in the region perhaps better than any other food group. The flavors of Mediterranean salads doesn't come from a bottle of commercially prepared dressing full of chemicals and other unfamiliar ingredients. Instead, they come from fresh vegetables and other good-for-you ingredients. What's more, you can customize your salads based on what's in season. If you crave something crunchy, you can top your salad with toasted pine nuts or pita chips instead of fat-laden carb-heavy croutons. And a salad doesn't have to even have lettuce in it. You can combine vegetables, fruits, nuts, barley, or bulgur wheat to make an amazingly healthy and flavorful salad without a lot of work.

Too often, people douse their salads with dressing, which adds a lot of unnecessary calories and really hides the flavor of the fresh vegetables. In the Mediterranean diet, however, the dressing is an accent to the flavor of the vegetables. It's usually light and bright and contains citrus or vinegar, which also helps in digestion. Most dressing bases start with extra-virgin olive oil, and are combined with, among other ingredients, a nice vinegar. Feel free to experiment with both and find the flavors you like best.

In This Chapter

- Fresh and flavorful salads
- Hearty, filling main dish salads
- Sensational side dish salads
- Light and tasty dressings

Tabbouleh Salad

In this satisfying salad, the vegetable, herb, and bulgur flavors combine to make this a salad you can enjoy almost any time of day as a main dish or a sensational side. The whole-grain bulgur wheat boosts the nutritional benefits, upping the protein content, which makes the salad very filling.

Yield:	Prep time:	Serving size:	
8 cups	1 hour	1 cup	
Each serving has:			
178 calories	14g fat	2g saturated fat	3g protein
13g carbohydrate	4g dietary fiber	0mg cholesterol	315mg sodium

$^1/_2$ cup bulgur wheat, grind #1

1 cup water

4 cups finely chopped fresh flat-leaf parsley, stems removed

3 medium tomatoes, finely diced

4 medium whole green onions, chopped

$^1/_2$ medium yellow onion, finely chopped

$^1/_4$ cup fresh mint, finely chopped

1 TB. dried mint

1 tsp. salt

$^1/_3$ cup fresh lemon juice

$^1/_2$ cup extra-virgin olive oil

$^1/_2$ tsp. cayenne

1. In a medium bowl, rinse bulgur wheat in water, pour off water, and let bulgur sit at room temperature for 30 minutes.

2. In a large bowl, combine flat-leaf parsley, tomatoes, green onions, yellow onion, fresh mint, and dried mint.

3. Add bulgur, salt, lemon juice, extra-virgin olive oil, and cayenne, and mix well.

4. Serve immediately, or store in the refrigerator to enjoy for 1 or 2 days.

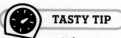 **TASTY TIP**

When using fresh herbs, be sure to rinse them very well before adding them to your dish to remove any dirt. To clean fresh herbs, cut off any large stems if necessary, place the leaves in a large bowl of cold water, and toss the herbs to remove as much dirt as possible. Remove the herbs from the water, drain in a colander, and repeat.

Fattoush Salad

This is a staple salad in the Mediterranean diet. It incorporates many colorful vegetables with a zesty garlic-herb dressing and boasts a crunchy pita chip topping. Top it with chicken or fish for an easy main dish.

Yield:	Prep time:	Serving size:	
12 cups	20 minutes	2 cups	
Each serving has:			
206 calories	10g fat	1g saturated fat	5g protein
26g carbohydrate	3g dietary fiber	0mg cholesterol	762mg sodium

1 large head romaine lettuce, chopped (3 cups)

$1/4$ medium head red cabbage, shredded (1 cup)

$1/2$ large orange bell pepper, ribs and seeds removed, and finely diced ($1/2$ cup)

$1/2$ large red bell pepper, ribs and seeds removed, and finely diced ($1/2$ cup)

$1/2$ large green bell pepper, ribs and seeds removed, and finely diced ($1/2$ cup)

1 large cucumber, diced (1 cup)

2 medium tomatoes, diced

$1/4$ cup red radishes, finely diced

1 large carrot, shredded ($1/4$ cup)

3 medium whole green onions, chopped

$1/2$ medium red onion, chopped

$1/2$ cup fresh flat-leaf parsley, finely chopped

1 tsp. dried mint

2 TB. sumac

$1^1/2$ tsp. salt

2 TB. minced garlic

$1/3$ cup fresh lemon juice

3 TB. apple cider vinegar

$1/4$ cup extra-virgin olive oil

2 cups pita chips, fried or baked

1. In a large bowl, combine romaine lettuce, red cabbage, orange bell pepper, red bell pepper, green bell pepper, cucumber, tomatoes, radishes, carrots, green onion, red onion, and flat-leaf parsley.

2. In a medium bowl, combine mint, sumac, salt, garlic, lemon juice, apple cider vinegar, and extra-virgin olive oil.

3. Pour dressing over vegetables, and toss until vegetables are well dressed.

4. Break pita chips into small, bite-size pieces, sprinkle on top of salad, and serve immediately.

Mediterranean Garden Salad

This is my go-to salad when I'm in a hurry but still craving a tasty salad. The nutty flavor of the tahini dressing complements the freshness of the vegetables and the crunchy pine nuts.

Yield:	Prep time:	Cook time:	Serving size:
8 cups	10 minutes	5 minutes	2 cups
Each serving has:			
314 calories	28g fat	3g saturated fat	6g protein
14g carbohydrate	4g dietary fiber	0mg cholesterol	327mg sodium

6 cups mixed greens

2 cups cherry tomatoes, halved

1 medium red onion, sliced ($^1/_2$ cup)

3 TB. tahini paste

3 TB. fresh lemon juice

3 TB. balsamic vinegar

3 TB. plus 1 tsp. extra-virgin olive oil

3 TB. water

$^1/_2$ tsp. salt

$^1/_2$ tsp. fresh ground black pepper

$^1/_2$ cup pine nuts

1. In a large bowl, add mixed greens, cherry tomatoes, and red onion.

2. In a small bowl, whisk together tahini paste, lemon juice, balsamic vinegar, 3 tablespoons extra-virgin olive oil, water, salt, and black pepper.

3. Preheat a small skillet over medium-low heat for 1 minute. Add remaining 1 teaspoon extra-virgin olive oil and pine nuts, and cook, stirring to toast evenly on all sides, for 4 minutes. Transfer pine nuts to a plate, and let cool for 2 minutes.

4. Pour dressing over vegetables, and toss to coat evenly. Top with toasted pine nuts, and serve immediately.

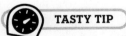 **TASTY TIP**

It's best to dress your salad right before serving it. Dressing it early wilts the vegetables and results in a soggy salad as the citrus and salt in the dressing break down the cell walls of the vegetables and draw out the moisture. Topping your salad with toasted nuts is a great way to omit carbs yet still have the satisfaction of something crunchy and flavorful on your salad.

Tomato and Cucumber Salad

This salad reminds me of summers in Michigan. My mom used to make this salad when it was hot outside and she didn't feel like cooking. It goes great with anything, even a cheese or hummus sandwich. The light combination of cucumbers, tomatoes, and herbs makes this salad very refreshing.

Yield:	**Prep time:**	**Serving size:**	
6 cups	10 minutes	2 cups	
Each serving has:			
234 calories	19g fat	3g saturated fat	3g protein
16g carbohydrate	4g dietary fiber	0mg cholesterol	404mg sodium

4 medium Persian cucumbers, diced

2 medium tomatoes, diced

1 medium white or red onion, chopped

$^1/_4$ cup flat-leaf parsley, finely chopped

3 TB. fresh mint, finely chopped

1 TB. minced garlic

$^1/_4$ cup fresh lemon juice

$^1/_4$ cup extra-virgin olive oil

$^1/_2$ tsp. salt

1. In a large bowl, combine Persian cucumbers, tomatoes, white onion, flat-leaf parsley, and mint.

2. In a small bowl, combine garlic, lemon juice, extra-virgin olive oil, and salt.

3. Pour dressing over vegetables, and toss until well dressed.

4. Serve immediately.

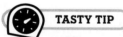 **TASTY TIP**

Always mix the dressing together in a separate bowl before adding it to the vegetables to avoid getting a mouthful of garlic or any other single dressing ingredient. If you're a lettuce lover, you can easily toss in any lettuce you like to this salad. If it's difficult to find Persian cucumbers, you can use any cucumber you can find.

Mediterranean Potato Salad

This version of potato salad is healthy and less fattening than traditional potato salad. The potatoes are roasted and then seasoned with an herb dressing that awakens your taste buds, while the citrus in the dressing helps lighten the starches from the potatoes. This salad is equally great for a cold winter evening or a hot summer afternoon.

Yield:	Prep time:	Cook time:	Serving size:
8 cups	20 minutes	25 minutes	2 cups
Each serving has:			
494 calories	31g fat	4g saturated fat	6g protein
49g carbohydrate	7g dietary fiber	0mg cholesterol	1,163mg sodium

2 lb. small red-skinned potatoes, washed and quartered

$^1/_2$ cup extra-virgin olive oil

1 tsp. salt

1 cup kalamata olives, pitted

$^1/_4$ cup capers, drained

2 TB. fresh thyme, chopped

2 whole green onions, chopped

$^1/_2$ cup fresh flat-leaf parsley, chopped

1 TB. lemon zest

1 TB. ground coriander seeds

3 TB. red wine vinegar

3 TB. fresh lemon juice

$^1/_2$ tsp. fresh ground black pepper

1. Preheat the oven to 450°F.

2. Place red-skinned potatoes on a baking sheet, drizzle with $^1/_4$ cup extra-virgin olive oil and $^1/_2$ teaspoon salt, and toss to coat evenly.

3. Bake potatoes for 25 minutes. Remove from the oven, and let cool on the baking sheet for 20 minutes.

4. In a large bowl, add potatoes, kalamata olives, capers, thyme, green onions, and flat-leaf parsley.

5. In a small bowl, whisk together lemon zest, ground coriander seeds, red wine vinegar, lemon juice, remaining $^1/_4$ cup extra-virgin olive oil, remaining $^1/_2$ teaspoon salt, and black pepper.

6. Pour dressing over potatoes, and toss to coat.

7. Serve immediately, or cover and refrigerate to enjoy for up to 3 days.

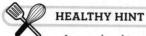 **HEALTHY HINT**

Leave the skin on your potatoes when making **Mediterranean Potato Salad**. Half the fiber found in potatoes is in the skin. Just be sure to wash your skin-on potatoes well before baking. I like to use a soft sponge with vegetable soap to help remove any excess dirt.

Roasted Beet Salad

Roasted beets have a wonderful sweet and earthy flavor, and combining them with the pungent flavor of the feta cheese awakens your taste buds. This zesty salad goes great with a piece of warm toasted Italian bread drizzled with olive oil.

Yield:	Prep time:	Cook time:	Serving size:
10 cups	20 minutes	40 minutes	2 cups
Each serving has:			
260 calories	18g fat	6g saturated fat	8g protein
19g carbohydrate	8g dietary fiber	27mg cholesterol	919mg sodium

6 medium fresh beets, root and stems ends trimmed, and rinsed

3 TB. water

1 whole red or yellow endive, finely sliced

1 medium red onion, finely sliced

$^1/_2$ cup red radishes, finely chopped

1 cup kalamata olives, pitted

2 TB. fresh chives, finely chopped

1 TB. fresh mint, finely chopped

1 TB. whole-grain mustard

1 TB. red wine vinegar

3 TB. fresh lemon juice

3 TB. extra-virgin olive oil

$^1/_2$ tsp. salt

$^1/_2$ tsp. fresh ground black pepper

1 cup feta cheese, crumbled

1. Preheat the oven to 400°F.

2. Place beets in a casserole dish, pour in water, cover the dish with aluminum foil, and bake for 40 minutes.

3. Remove beets from the oven, remove aluminum foil, and place beets on a plate to cool completely.

4. After beets have cooled, remove the skin and cut beets into $^1/_2$-inch cubes.

5. In a large bowl, add beets, red endive, red onion, radishes, kalamata olives, chives, and mint.

6. In a small bowl, whisk together whole-grain mustard, red wine vinegar, lemon juice, extra-virgin olive oil, salt, and black pepper.

7. Pour dressing over vegetables, and lightly toss. Top with crumbled feta cheese, and serve immediately.

 HEALTHY HINT

Beets contain betalains, which contain antioxidants, anti-inflammatories, and detoxifiers. Beets are often used to make pickled turnips fuchsia in color while still providing healthy benefits.

Quinoa Salad

This great one-dish-meal salad is loaded with protein and vegetables. The nutty, earthy flavor of the quinoa combines well with the chickpeas and the zesty dressing to satisfy your taste buds.

Yield:	Prep time:	Cook time:	Serving size:
6 cups	10 minutes	20 minutes	2 cups
Each serving has:			
468 calories	22g fat	3g saturated fat	12g protein
58g carbohydrate	10g dietary fiber	0mg cholesterol	758mg sodium

2 cups red quinoa

4 cups water

1 (15-oz.) can chickpeas, drained

1 medium red onion, chopped ($^1/_2$ cup)

3 TB. fresh mint leaves, finely chopped

$^1/_4$ cup extra-virgin olive oil

3 TB. fresh lemon juice

$^1/_2$ tsp. salt

$^1/_2$ tsp. fresh ground black pepper

1. In a medium saucepan over medium-high heat, bring red quinoa and water to a boil. Cover, reduce heat to low, and cook for 20 minutes or until water is absorbed and quinoa is tender. Let cool.

2. In a large bowl, add quinoa, chickpeas, red onion, and mint.

3. In a small bowl, whisk together extra-virgin olive oil, lemon juice, salt, and black pepper.

4. Pour dressing over quinoa mixture, and stir well to combine.

5. Serve immediately, or refrigerate and enjoy for up to 2 or 3 days.

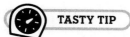 **TASTY TIP**

Unlike salads with a leafy base, Quinoa Salad holds up to a citrus dressing. I like making the salad ahead of time and then enjoying it for a few days later. Just keep it covered and refrigerated, and the flavor will continue to get better over time.

Warm Mediterranean Salad

With the smoky flavor of the grilled vegetables, the nutty barley, and the tangy goat cheese, this salad is guaranteed to make you happy.

Yield:	Prep time:	Cook time:	Serving size:
8 cups	4^1/$_2$ hours	1 hour, 9 minutes	2 cups

Each serving has:			
573 calories	25g fat	8g saturated fat	23g protein
74g carbohydrate	21g dietary fiber	23mg cholesterol	952mg sodium

1 cup hulled barley	^{1}/$_4$ cup fresh parsley, chopped
2 cups water	4 TB. extra-virgin olive oil
12 asparagus stalks	3 TB. balsamic vinegar
1 whole red bell pepper	^{1}/$_2$ tsp. salt
2 cups water	^{1}/$_2$ tsp. fresh ground black pepper
8 canned or jarred artichoke hearts, halved	4 oz. goat cheese
1 cup cherry tomatoes, halved	^{1}/$_2$ cup panko breadcrumbs

1. In a medium bowl, soak hulled barley in warm water to cover for 4 hours. Drain.

2. In a medium saucepan over medium heat, bring barley and 2 cups water to a boil. Cover, reduce heat to low, and cook for 40 minutes or until water is absorbed and barley is tender. Let cool.

3. Preheat a grill top or grill to medium.

4. Grill asparagus on all sides for about 5 minutes. Chop asparagus into 2-inch pieces, and place in a large bowl.

5. Grill red bell pepper on all sides for about 20 minutes or until charred. Immediately place pepper onto a plate, cover with plastic wrap, and set aside to cool for 10 minutes.

6. Peel skin off red pepper (it's okay if it doesn't all come off), and remove the stem, ribs, and seeds. Slice pepper into ^{1}/$_4$-inch strips, and add to the large bowl.

7. Add barley to asparagus and red bell pepper. Add artichoke hearts, cherry tomatoes, parsley, 2 tablespoons extra-virgin olive oil, balsamic vinegar, salt, and black pepper, and toss to combine.

8. Cut goat cheese into 4 equal pieces, and coat all sides of cheese with panko breadcrumbs.

9. Preheat a small skillet over low heat, and add remaining 2 tablespoons extra-virgin olive oil. Add panko-coated goat cheese slices, and brown on both sides for about 2 minutes per side.

10. To serve, place $^1/_4$ of salad mixture on a plate, top with 1 goat cheese slice, and serve immediately.

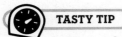 **TASTY TIP**

> To save a bit of time as you make this salad, you can prep the barley ahead of time and store it in a container in the refrigerator. Then, when you're ready to make this salad, you can just toss it in.

Mediterranean Pasta Salad

This is a mayonnaise-free pasta salad. The traditional mayo dressing is replaced with a tangy vinegar-herb dressing with a little kick, thanks to the crushed red pepper flakes.

Yield:	Prep time:	Cook time:	Serving size:
10 cups	10 minutes	8 minutes	1 cup
Each serving has:			
320 calories	22g fat	5g saturated fat	10g protein
20g carbohydrate	1g dietary fiber	37mg cholesterol	1,499mg sodium

1 TB. plus 1 tsp. salt

1 lb. bag farfalle pasta

1 large tomato, chopped

2 cups flat-leaf parsley, finely chopped

4 whole green onions, finely chopped

$^1/_4$ cup fresh basil, finely chopped

1 medium red bell pepper, ribs and seeds removed, and finely diced

1 cup kalamata olives, pitted

1 tsp. dried oregano

1 tsp. dried mint

1 tsp. crushed red pepper flakes

1 tsp. dried thyme

1 tsp. fresh ground black pepper

$^1/_4$ cup balsamic vinegar

$^1/_4$ cup white balsamic vinegar

$^1/_2$ cup extra-virgin olive oil

10 oz. fresh mini mozzarella balls

1. Bring a large pot of water to a boil over high heat. Season with 1 tablespoon salt, add far-falle pasta, cook for 8 minutes, and drain.

2. In a large bowl, toss together pasta, tomato, flat-leaf parsley, green onions, basil, red bell pepper, and kalamata olives.

3. Add oregano, mint, crushed red pepper flakes, thyme, remaining 1 teaspoon salt, black pepper, balsamic vinegar, white balsamic vinegar, and extra-virgin olive oil, and toss until everything is well coated.

4. Top pasta with mozzarella balls and serve immediately, or cover and refrigerate to enjoy for 2 or 3 days.

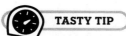 **TASTY TIP**

You can replace the mozzarella cheese with 4 ounces of crumbled goat cheese or $^1/_2$ cup grated Parmesan cheese if you like.

Spinach Salad

This light and refreshing salad will change the way you think about spinach. The tangy dressing offsets the leafy flavor of the spinach quite nicely.

Yield:	Prep time:	Serving size:	
8 cups	10 minutes	2 cups	
Each serving has:			
133 calories	11g fat	2g saturated fat	2g protein
9g carbohydrate	2g dietary fiber	0mg cholesterol	332mg sodium

6 cups baby spinach, washed	1 TB. apple cider vinegar
2 medium tomatoes, chopped	1 TB. minced garlic
1 medium red onion, sliced	1 TB. sumac
$^1/_4$ cup fresh lemon juice	1 tsp. dried mint
3 TB. extra-virgin olive oil	$^1/_2$ tsp. salt

1. In a large bowl, add spinach, tomatoes, and red onions.

2. In a small bowl, whisk together lemon juice, extra-virgin olive oil, apple cider vinegar, garlic, sumac, mint, and salt.

3. Pour dressing over spinach mixture, toss to coat, and serve immediately.

Greek Salad

When I think of Mediterranean salad, the first thing that comes to mind is a Greek salad. I love the crunchy cucumbers with the smooth feta and the herb dressing. A bowl of this salad with some grilled chicken just makes me happy.

Yield:	Prep time:	Serving size:	
8 cups	10 minutes	2 cups	
Each serving has:			
443 calories	36g fat	8g saturated fat	8g protein
21g carbohydrate	4g dietary fiber	33mg cholesterol	1,580mg sodium

8 large leaves romaine lettuce, chopped

2 medium tomatoes, diced large

3 medium Persian cucumbers, sliced

1 medium red onion, thinly sliced

1 medium green bell pepper, ribs and seeds removed, and thinly sliced

$^1/_4$ cup extra-virgin olive oil

3 TB. fresh lemon juice

1 TB. red wine vinegar

1 TB. minced garlic

$^1/_2$ tsp. salt

1 TB. dried oregano

1 cup kalamata olives, pitted

1 cup feta cheese, crumbled

1. In a large bowl, add romaine lettuce, tomatoes, Persian cucumbers, red onion, and green bell pepper.

2. In a small bowl, whisk together extra-virgin olive oil, lemon juice, red wine vinegar, garlic, salt, and oregano.

3. Pour dressing over lettuce mixture, and toss to coat.

4. Top salad with kalamata olives and feta, and serve immediately.

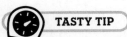 **TASTY TIP**

If you don't like feta cheese, you can definitely replace it with a cheese of your choice. Goat cheese or fresh mozzarella also work well with this recipe.

Lentil Salad

I love this salad because I know it's so healthy. The lentils make it very hearty and filling, so it can be served as a main course salad or as a side for grilled chicken or fish.

Yield:	Prep time:	Cook time:	Serving size:
6 cups	30 minutes	25 minutes	1 cup

Each serving has:			
188 calories	10g fat	1g saturated fat	7g protein
20g carbohydrate	5g dietary fiber	0mg cholesterol	348mg sodium

2 cups green or brown lentils, picked over and rinsed	$^1/_2$ cup fresh flat-leaf parsley, finely chopped
1 bay leaf	1 TB. fresh mint
4 cups water	$^1/_4$ cup extra-virgin olive oil
$^1/_4$ medium white onion, finely chopped	$^1/_4$ cup fresh lemon juice
2 medium tomatoes, finely diced	1 tsp. salt
3 medium Persian cucumbers, finely diced	1 tsp. dried mint
$^1/_2$ medium red onion, finely chopped	$^1/_2$ tsp. cayenne

1. In a large saucepan over medium heat, combine green lentils, bay leaf, water, and white onion. Bring to a boil, reduce heat to medium-low, and cook for 25 minutes or until lentils are tender. Drain, remove onion and bay leaf, and set lentils aside to cool.

2. In a large bowl, add cooked lentils, tomatoes, Persian cucumbers, red onion, flat-leaf parsley, and fresh mint.

3. In a small bowl, whisk together extra-virgin olive oil, lemon juice, salt, dried mint, and cayenne.

4. Pour dressing over lentil mix, and toss to coat evenly.

5. Serve immediately, or cover and refrigerate to enjoy for 1 or 2 days.

Bean Salad

I like to think of this salad as a protein salad because it's chock full of protein and lots of fiber. The citrus dressing lightens the heaviness of the beans.

Yield:	Prep time:	Serving size:	
5 cups	10 minutes	1 cup	
Each serving has:			
181 calories	9g fat	1g saturated fat	7g protein
21g carbohydrate	4g dietary fiber	0mg cholesterol	248mg sodium

1 (15-oz.) can cannellini beans, drained	3 TB. fresh thyme
1 (15-oz.) can fava beans, drained	1 TB. lemon zest
1 medium red bell pepper, ribs and seeds removed, and finely chopped	3 TB. extra-virgin olive oil
	3 TB. fresh lemon juice
$^1/_2$ medium white onion, finely chopped	1 TB. apple cider vinegar
	1 tsp. minced garlic
$^1/_2$ cup fresh flat-leaf parsley, finely chopped	$^1/_2$ tsp. salt

1. In a large bowl, combine cannellini beans, fava beans, red bell pepper, white onion, flat-leaf parsley, and thyme.

2. In a small bowl, whisk together lemon zest, extra-virgin olive oil, lemon juice, apple cider vinegar, garlic, and salt.

3. Pour dressing over bean mixture, and toss to coat evenly.

4. Serve immediately, or cover and refrigerate to enjoy for another 1 or 2 days.

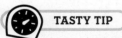 **TASTY TIP**

Bean salads hold up really well to dressings, so making this dish in advance is a great idea—you can enjoy it for a few days after as well. The flavor actually develops more the longer it sits, so it will taste even better.

Fig Salad

Figs are so sweet and hearty, they always satisfy my sweet tooth. Here, they're combined with the earthy flavor of bulgur and spicy arugula.

Yield:	Prep time:	Cook time:	Serving size:
10 cups	40 minutes	15 minutes	2 cups

Each serving has:			
440 calories	24g fat	3g saturated fat	7g protein
56g carbohydrate	9g dietary fiber	0mg cholesterol	249mg sodium

2 cups dried figs

2 cups hot water

2 cups water

1 cup bulgur wheat, grind #2

6 cups fresh arugula

1 cup plain walnuts

2 TB. honey

3 TB. red wine vinegar

3 TB. extra-virgin olive oil

$^1/_2$ tsp. salt

$^1/_2$ tsp. fresh ground black pepper

1. In a medium bowl, add figs. Pour hot water over figs, set aside to soak for 30 minutes, and drain. Cut figs into quarters.

2. In a large saucepan over medium heat, bring 2 cups water to a boil. Add bulgur wheat, reduce heat to low, cover, and cook for 15 minutes or until all of water is absorbed. Fluff with a fork, and let cool.

3. In a large bowl, add arugula, figs, bulgur wheat, and walnuts.

4. In a small bowl, whisk together honey, red wine vinegar, extra-virgin olive oil, salt, and black pepper.

5. Pour dressing over arugula mixture, and toss to coat.

6. Serve immediately.

Watermelon Salad

This salad brings me memories of hot summer nights, sitting on the porch with my dad, and eating watermelon and feta cheese. The sweetness of the watermelon and the saltiness of the feta complement each other nicely.

Yield:	Prep time:	Serving size:	
10 cups	10 minutes	1 cup	
Each serving has:			
205 calories	7g fat	2g saturated fat	4g protein
35g carbohydrate	2g dietary fiber	10mg cholesterol	133mg sodium

1 (5-lb.) seedless watermelon	3 TB. extra-virgin olive oil
4 oz. feta cheese, crumbled	2 TB. fresh lemon juice
3 TB. fresh mint, finely chopped	

1. Scoop watermelon into balls, or cut into $1/_2$-inch cubes.

2. In a large bowl, add watermelon and feta cheese.

3. In a small bowl, combine mint, extra-virgin olive oil, and lemon juice.

4. Pour dressing over watermelon and feta, and toss gently.

5. Serve immediately.

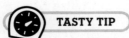 **TASTY TIP**

Watermelon is crispy and refreshing ... but not when it's soggy. When serving or prepping watermelon, cut it right before serving to ensure the best taste and texture.

Mediterranean Dressing

I always keep this dressing in my refrigerator for whenever I want to throw together a quick salad. It has all-around flavor that's great for any salad mix.

Yield:	Prep time:	Serving size:	
about 1²/₃ cups	5 minutes	2 tablespoons	
Each serving has:			
151 calories	17g fat	2g saturated fat	0g protein
1g carbohydrate	0g dietary fiber	0mg cholesterol	180mg sodium

1 cup extra-virgin olive oil	1 tsp. salt
¹/₃ cup fresh lemon juice	2 TB. sumac
3 TB. apple cider vinegar	1 TB. dried mint
2 TB. minced garlic	

1. Add extra-virgin olive oil, lemon juice, apple cider vinegar, garlic, salt, sumac, and mint to a dressing bottle or glass jar. Cover and shake until well combined.

2. Refrigerate for up to 2 weeks.

 MEDITERRANEAN MORSEL

Making your own salad dressing is a great way to control the amount of calories it contains. And experimenting with different dried herbs or spices in dressings is a great way to create new flavors for your salad, roasted vegetables, or meats.

Super Soups

Mediterranean soups are chock full of wonderful ingredients. And these aren't thin soups—the hearty soups in this chapter make a complete meal in a single bowl. Many contain beans or meat; fresh vegetables; and complex carbohydrates in the form of wheat, barley, or noodles. In addition, the herbs and spices provide so much flavor, they eliminate the need for fats or heavy creams.

Mediterranean soups contain many of the nutrients and elements you need in a balanced meal. Some have lentils that are full of protein and iron and keep you feeling full. Others are loaded with meat or chicken—excellent sources of protein—with an abundance of vegetables.

These soups also enable you to cook once and eat for a few days. They keep well when refrigerated.

Best of all, you can use whatever vegetables you like when they're in season. Soups have traditionally been made with what's available in the pantry and garden. If you have lentils, green wheat, or barley, plus a few vegetables, you can make a great-tasting soup. And don't think of soups as just for cold weather fare. They're great all year round.

In This Chapter

- Rich and flavorful soups
- Hearty meals in a bowl
- Soups to warm you from the inside

Beef and Vegetable Soup

This rich and hearty soup boasts tender chunks of beef seasoned with herbs and vegetables. It goes great with a toasted piece of bread.

Yield:	Prep time:	Cook time:	Serving size:
12 cups	30 minutes	45 minutes	2 cups

Each serving has:			
527 calories	22g fat	5g saturated fat	42g protein
40g carbohydrate	6g dietary fiber	96mg cholesterol	1,136mg sodium

2 lb. boneless beef chuck, cut into
   $^1/_2$-in. cubes

2 medium yellow onions, chopped

3 bay leaves

2 tsp. salt

12 cups water

1 (15-oz.) can tomato sauce

3 TB. tomato paste

1 tsp. dried oregano

4 medium carrots, chopped

2 medium zucchini, diced

1 cup fresh or frozen corn

5 TB. extra-virgin olive oil

1 cup vermicelli noodles

$^1/_2$ cup fresh parsley, chopped

$^1/_2$ tsp. ground black pepper

1. In a pressure cooker pot over medium heat, combine beef, half of yellow onions, bay leaves, salt, and water. Bring to a simmer, uncovered, and skim off any foam that rises to the top.

2. Add pressure cooker lid, reduce heat to low, and cook for 20 minutes.

3. Release steam from the pressure cooker, and set aside to cool for at least 20 minutes before removing the lid.

4. Remove and discard bay leaves.

5. Return the pot to medium-low heat. Add tomato sauce, tomato paste, and oregano, and bring to a simmer.

6. Add carrots, zucchini, and corn; stir; and continue to simmer.

7. In a small saucepan over medium heat, heat 3 tablespoons extra-virgin olive oil. Add remaining half of yellow onions, and sauté for 5 minutes. Add to soup.

8. In the same small saucepan over medium heat, heat remaining 2 tablespoons extra-virgin olive oil. Add vermicelli noodles, and cook, stirring to brown evenly, for about 3 minutes. Add to the soup, stir, and cook for 10 minutes.

9. Add parsley and black pepper to soup, stir, and serve.

Chicken Soup

Chicken soup is a classic remedy for a cold, but you don't have to be ill to enjoy this hearty chicken soup. The subtle Mediterranean flavors give it a lovely face-lift.

Yield:	Prep time:	Cook time:	Serving size:
12 cups	30 minutes	1 hour, 10 minutes	2 cups

Each serving has:			
415 calories	18g fat	3g saturated fat	24g protein
40g carbohydrate	6g dietary fiber	64mg cholesterol	692mg sodium

1 (3-lb.) whole chicken	5 medium carrots, chopped
3 bay leaves	3 medium stalks celery, chopped
5 whole allspice	5 TB. extra-virgin olive oil
1 (2-in.) cinnamon stick	$^1/_2$ medium yellow onion, chopped
$^1/_2$ medium yellow onion, sliced	1 cup vermicelli noodles
$1^1/_2$ tsp. salt	1 large potato, peeled and diced
10 cups water	$^1/_2$ cup fresh parsley, chopped

1. In a large pot over high heat, combine chicken, bay leaves, allspice, cinnamon stick, sliced yellow onion, 1 teaspoon salt, and water. Bring to a boil, reduce heat to medium-low, and simmer for 40 minutes, skimming any foam that rises to the top.

2. Remove chicken from the pot, and set aside to cool enough to handle. Pick chicken apart, removing skin and bones, and cut into bite-size pieces.

3. Strain broth, discard solids, and return broth and boneless chicken pieces to the pot over medium-low heat.

4. Add carrots and celery, and cook for 10 minutes.

5. In a small saucepan over medium heat, heat 3 tablespoons extra-virgin olive oil. Add chopped yellow onion, and sauté for 5 minutes. Add to the pot.

6. In the same small saucepan over medium heat, heat remaining 2 tablespoons extra-virgin olive oil. Add vermicelli noodles, and cook, stirring to brown evenly, for 3 minutes.

7. Add toasted vermicelli noodles and diced potato to the pot, and cook for 10 minutes.

8. Add parsley, remove from heat, and serve.

Pumpkin Soup

This pumpkin soup defines the flavors of fall, with a Mediterranean twist. The smooth flavor of the pumpkin with the warm spices make this soup the perfect remedy for a chilly day.

Yield:	Prep time:	Cook time:	Serving size:
12 cups	20 minutes	1 hour, 11 minutes	2 cups

Each serving has:			
333 calories	21g fat	7g saturated fat	10g protein
30g carbohydrate	8g dietary fiber	27mg cholesterol	1,210mg sodium

1 medium sugar pumpkin

1 medium potato, peeled and cut into 1-in. cubes

3 TB. extra-virgin olive oil

4 medium carrots

2 medium stalks celery

$1/2$ medium white onion, chopped

1 tsp. salt

3 TB. fresh sage, chopped

6 cups chicken or vegetable stock

1 tsp. ground cumin

1 tsp. ground coriander

$1/2$ tsp. turmeric

$1/2$ tsp. ground nutmeg

$1/2$ tsp. cinnamon

2 tsp. sugar

$1/2$ cup heavy cream

$1/3$ cup sunflower seeds

1. Preheat the oven to 450°F.

2. Cut sugar pumpkin in half, and remove seeds. Place pumpkin cut side down on a baking sheet, and bake for 40 minutes.

3. Meanwhile, in a small saucepan over medium heat, boil potato in water to cover for about 7 minutes or until tender. Drain and set aside.

4. Scoop out pumpkin flesh and set aside.

5. In a large pot over medium heat, heat extra-virgin olive oil. Add carrots, celery, white onion, and salt, and sauté, stirring occasionally, for 10 minutes.

6. Add sage, and cook for 4 more minutes.

7. Add chicken stock, and cook for 5 minutes.

8. Add pumpkin and potato, and using a handheld immersion blender or in a food processor fitted with a chopping blade, blend mixture for 1 or 2 minutes or until smooth.

9. Add cumin, coriander, turmeric, nutmeg, cinnamon, and sugar. Reduce heat to medium-low, and cook for 10 minutes.

10. Add heavy cream, and remove from heat.

11. In a small saucepan over medium heat, toast sunflower seeds for 2 minutes or until golden brown.

12. Serve immediately, topped with toasted sunflower seeds.

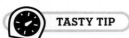 **TASTY TIP**

If you can't find a sugar pumpkin, you can use 4 cups canned pumpkin purée instead.

Yellow Lentil Soup

This is a very easy lentil soup recipe, you can add as many or as few vegetables as you like. The earthy flavor of the lentils, combined with the array of spices, awakens your taste buds with each bite.

Yield:	Prep time:	Cook time:	Serving size:
12 cups	20 minutes	55 minutes	2 cups
Each serving has:			
150 calories	8g fat	1g saturated fat	4g protein
18g carbohydrate	4g dietary fiber	0mg cholesterol	812mg sodium

1 cup red/orange lentils, picked over and rinsed

1/2 cup long-grain rice

10 cups water

2 tsp. salt

3 TB. extra-virgin olive oil

1 medium yellow onion, chopped

4 medium carrots, diced

1 tsp. turmeric

1 tsp. cumin

1 tsp. coriander

1/2 tsp. ground black pepper

1 cup fresh parsley, finely chopped

1 medium lemon, quartered (optional)

1. In a large pot over medium-low heat, combine red/orange lentils, long-grain rice, water, and salt. Cook, stirring occasionally, for 40 minutes.

2. In a small saucepan over medium-low heat, heat extra-virgin olive oil. Add yellow onion, and sauté, stirring occasionally, for 5 minutes.

3. Add carrots, sautéed onions, turmeric, cumin, coriander, and black pepper to the large pot; stir; and cook for 10 minutes.

4. Stir in parsley, and remove the pot from heat.

5. Serve soup with lemon wedge to squeeze onto soup (if using).

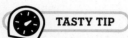 **TASTY TIP**

This is one of my go-to soups because it requires very little work and very few ingredients. Best of all, it stores well. You can refrigerate it for up to 1 week.

Hearty Brown Lentil Soup

This brown lentil soup is warming and filling. Mini meatballs, potatoes, and brown lentils come together to deliver a well-rounded meal in a bowl.

Yield:	Prep time:	Cook time:	Serving size:
12 cups	20 minutes	1 hour, 20 minutes	2 cups
Each serving has:			
282 calories	11g fat	2g saturated fat	15g protein
32g carbohydrate	7g dietary fiber	23mg cholesterol	802mg sodium

2 cups brown lentils, picked over
    and rinsed

14 cups water

2 tsp. salt

$^1/_4$ cup long-grain rice

$^1/_2$ lb. lean ground beef

1 tsp. ground black pepper

3 TB. extra-virgin olive oil

1 medium yellow onion, chopped

1 TB. cumin

$^1/_2$ cup fresh parsley, chopped

2 medium potatoes, peeled and
    medium diced

1. In a large pot over medium-low heat, combine brown lentils, water, and 1 teaspoon salt. Bring to a simmer, and cook, stirring occasionally, for 1 hour.

2. Remove the pot from heat. Using a handheld immersion blender or in a food processor fitted with a chopping blade, blend lentils for 1 or 2 minutes or until smooth. If desired, strain soup to remove any pulp from lentil skins.

3. Set the pot over low heat, add long-grain rice, and cook, stirring occasionally to stop rice from clumping, for 10 minutes.

4. In a small bowl, combine ground beef, $^1/_2$ teaspoon salt, and $^1/_2$ teaspoon black pepper. Form mixture into about 20 to 30 ($^1/_2$-inch) meatballs.

5. In a small skillet over medium heat, cook meatballs for 6 minutes, turning over every 2 minutes until browned on all sides. Add cooked meatballs to soup.

6. In the small skillet, heat extra-virgin olive oil. Add yellow onion, and sauté for 5 minutes. Add onion to soup.

7. Add remaining $^1/_2$ teaspoon salt, remaining $^1/_2$ teaspoon black pepper, cumin, parsley, and potatoes to soup, and stir to combine. Cook for 5 minutes.

8. Remove from heat, and serve.

MEDITERRANEAN MORSEL

Sometimes tiny pebbles or rocks or pieces of grain are included with the dry lentils. To ensure you remove all these stray bits, pick over the lentils. Pour the lentils onto a plate, and using your fingers, pick through the lentils, moving them around to be sure no pebbles or pieces of grain are in the mix.

Lentil and Swiss Chard Soup

My mom would make this soup as an alternative to chicken soup when I was sick because she said "It has so much vitamins." She was right! This soup has a very light taste, the Swiss chard and lemon flavors are refreshing, and the lentils fill you up.

Yield:	Prep time:	Cook time:	Serving size:
12 cups	20 minutes	1 hour	2 cups
Each serving has:			
241 calories	10g fat	1g saturated fat	9g protein
33g carbohydrate	7g dietary fiber	0mg cholesterol	1,043mg sodium

12 cups water

2 tsp. salt

$1^1/_2$ cups brown or green lentils, picked over and rinsed

6 medium garlic cloves, finely chopped

2 lb. Swiss chard (about 2 bunches), washed and chopped

2 medium yellow onions, chopped

4 TB. extra-virgin olive oil

1 large potato, peeled and diced

$^1/_2$ tsp. ground black pepper

$^1/_4$ cup fresh lemon juice

1. In a large pot over medium heat, combine water, 1 teaspoon salt, and brown lentils. Simmer for 30 minutes.

2. Add remaining 1 teaspoon salt, garlic, Swiss chard, and half of onions; stir; and simmer for 20 minutes.

3. In a small pan over medium heat, heat extra-virgin olive oil. Add remaining yellow onions, and sauté for 5 minutes. Add onions to the large pot.

4. Add potato, black pepper, and lemon juice to the pot, and simmer for 5 minutes.

5. Serve warm.

Freekeh Soup

Freekeh is a smoked green wheat that contains an abundance of nutrients, including protein and fiber, and has a low glycemic index. The smoked green wheat gives this dish an unbelievable hearty and earthy flavor.

Yield:	Prep time:	Cook time:	Serving size:
10 cups	30 minutes	1 hour	2 cups

Each serving has:			
599 calories	24g fat	6g saturated fat	44g protein
52g carbohydrate	11g dietary fiber	109mg cholesterol	1,198mg sodium

2 lb. boneless beef chuck, cut into ¹/₂-in. cubes

2 medium yellow onions, chopped

3 bay leaves

2 tsp. salt

10 cups water

1 cup freekeh

3 TB. extra-virgin olive oil

1 TB. garlic, minced

1 (15-oz.) can chickpeas, drained

2 cups kale, washed and chopped

1 tsp. ground coriander

¹/₂ tsp. ground white pepper

1. In a pressure cooker pot over medium heat, combine beef chuck, half of yellow onions, bay leaves, salt, and water. Bring to a simmer, skimming any foam that rises to the top.

2. Add pressure cooker lid, reduce heat to low, and cook for 20 minutes.

3. Release steam from the pressure cooker, and set aside to cool for at least 20 minutes before removing the lid.

4. Remove and discard bay leaves.

5. Stir in freekeh, and simmer for 20 minutes.

6. In a small pan over medium heat, heat extra-virgin olive oil. Add remaining half of yellow onions and garlic, and sauté, stirring occasionally, for 5 minutes.

7. Add sautéed onions and garlic to the pot, and simmer for 5 minutes.

8. Add chickpeas, kale, coriander, and white pepper to the pot, and simmer for 10 more minutes.

9. Serve warm.

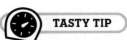 **TASTY TIP**

If you like lamb, you can replace the beef chuck in this recipe with lamb shank.

Barley and Chicken Soup

Barley has many uses, one of which is to make a wonderful chicken soup. I like to use hulled barley rather than pearl barley because it has more nutrients and a nuttier flavor.

Yield:	Prep time:	Cook time:	Serving size:
10 cups	4^1/$_2$ hours	1 hour, 2 minutes	2 cups

Each serving has:			
410 calories	16g fat	2g saturated fat	30g protein
37g carbohydrate	8g dietary fiber	45mg cholesterol	1,646mg sodium

1 cup hulled barley	2 medium carrots, chopped
2 cups warm water	2 TB. fresh thyme
5 TB. extra-virgin olive oil	1 tsp. salt
2 (6- to 8-oz.) boneless skinless chicken breasts, cut into ^{1}/$_2$-in. cubes	10 cups low-sodium chicken or vegetable broth
2 medium whole leeks, chopped	^{1}/$_2$ tsp. ground black pepper

1. In a medium bowl, soak hulled barley in warm water for 4 hours. Drain. (You can do this in advance.)

2. In a large pot over medium heat, heat 3 tablespoons extra-virgin olive oil. Add chicken, and cook, turning chicken over to brown evenly, for 7 minutes. Remove chicken from the pot, and set aside.

3. In the pot, heat remaining 2 tablespoons extra-virgin olive oil. Add leeks, carrots, and thyme, and cook, stirring occasionally, for 5 minutes.

4. Add drained barley, salt, and chicken broth to the pot, cover, and simmer over low heat for 40 minutes or until barley is tender.

5. Add cooked chicken and black pepper, and simmer for 10 minutes.

6. Serve warm.

Soothing Stews

Soups and stews are often grouped in the same category, but they are actually two very different dishes.

Many times, stews are a bit thicker with less broth. They're also very hearty; usually contain vegetables and a type of protein; and are often served with a grain like rice, bulgur pilaf, or even bread. If you're a vegetarian, the meat or protein can easily be omitted and replaced with more vegetables. A good-tasting broth is ideal to have on hand for any stew because it adds to the dish's flavor.

Stews are great for lunch or for dinner. Because they're so flavorful and well rounded, they can satisfy your hunger whether it's the middle of the day or after a long day at work.

Stews are very common along the Mediterranean because they're economical. Composed mostly of vegetables and a sauce with some protein, a pot of stew can feed a family for a day or two when served with a grain.

In This Chapter

- Hearty and warming stews
- Meal-worthy stews
- Vegetable-rich stews

Ghallaba Stew

This chicken stew boasts an array of fresh vegetables and vibrant tomato sauce. It's fantastic on its own or with a bowl of pasta or rice.

Yield:	Prep time:	Cook time:	Serving size:
10 cups	20 minutes	30 minutes	2 cups

Each serving has:			
286 calories	13g fat	2g saturated fat	25g protein
20g carbohydrate	5g dietary fiber	51mg cholesterol	1,563mg sodium

4 TB. extra-virgin olive oil

2 (8-oz.) boneless, skinless chicken breasts, cut into $^1/_2$-in. cubes

1 large red onion, chopped

$^1/_2$ large yellow bell pepper, ribs and seeds removed, and chopped

$^1/_2$ large red bell pepper, ribs and seeds removed, and chopped

$^1/_2$ large green bell pepper, ribs and seeds removed, and chopped

1 cup crimini mushrooms, sliced

3 large carrots, sliced

$1^1/_2$ tsp. salt

3 TB. minced garlic

3 cups plain tomato sauce

2 cups water

1 tsp. paprika

1 tsp. cayenne

1 tsp. ground black pepper

$^1/_2$ cup fresh parsley, finely chopped

1 TB. *sumac*

1. In a large, 3-quart pot over medium heat, heat extra-virgin olive oil. Add chicken, and cook for 5 minutes.

2. Add red onion, yellow bell pepper, red bell pepper, green bell pepper, crimini mushrooms, carrots, and salt, and cook for 5 minutes.

3. Add garlic, tomato sauce, water, paprika, cayenne, black pepper, and parsley. Stir and simmer for 10 minutes.

4. Serve warm with a sprinkle of sumac and a side of pasta or rice.

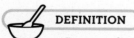

DEFINITION

Sumac is the fruit of a flowering plant that's dried and ground. It has a tart, tangy flavor.

Eggplant Stew

This is the perfect warm and filling winter stew, loaded with tender, juicy vegetables and a smooth tomato sauce.

Yield:	Prep time:	Cook time:	Serving size:
8 cups	20 minutes	35 minutes	1 cup

Each serving has:			
209 calories	6g fat	1g saturated fat	5g protein
37g carbohydrate	13g dietary fiber	0mg cholesterol	623mg sodium

3 TB. extra-virgin olive oil	1 large tomato, diced
1 medium white onion, chopped	1 (16-oz.) can tomato sauce
2 large carrots, sliced diagonally	1 tsp. garlic powder
4 medium Italian eggplant, trimmed and diced	1 tsp. paprika
	$1^1/_2$ tsp. salt
2 large potatoes, peeled and diced	1 cup fresh cilantro, chopped

1. In a 3-quart pot over medium heat, heat extra-virgin olive oil. Add white onion and carrots, and cook for 5 minutes.

2. Add Italian eggplant and potatoes, and cook for 7 minutes.

3. Add tomato, and cook for 3 minutes.

4. Add tomato sauce, garlic powder, paprika, and salt, and simmer, stirring occasionally, for 15 minutes.

5. Stir in cilantro, and cook for 5 more minutes.

6. Serve with brown rice.

Jew's Mallow Stew (*Mulukhiya*)

This recipe is very popular in the countries that border the Mediterranean on the South. It's a stew made with chicken and mallow leaves with refreshing cilantro and lemon.

Yield:	Prep time:	Cook time:	Serving size:
8 cups	30 minutes	2 hours	1 cup

Each serving has:			
204 calories	17g fat	3g saturated fat	6g protein
8g carbohydrate	2g dietary fiber	14mg cholesterol	596mg sodium

2 whole chicken thighs, including drumstick	6 cups rehydrated *Jew's mallow leaves*, drained
1 (2-in.) cinnamon stick	1 large yellow onion, chopped
2 bay leaves	6 TB. minced garlic
8 cups water	1 cup fresh cilantro, finely chopped
2 tsp. salt	$^1/_2$ tsp. cayenne
$^1/_2$ cup extra-virgin olive oil	$^1/_2$ cup fresh lemon juice

1. In a large pot over medium heat, combine chicken thighs, cinnamon stick, bay leaves, water, and 1 teaspoon salt. Cook for 30 minutes. Skim off any foam that comes to the top.

2. Meanwhile, in another large pot over medium heat, heat $^1/_4$ cup extra-virgin olive oil. Add Jew's mallow leaves, and cook, tossing leaves, for 10 minutes. Remove leaves, and set aside.

3. Reduce heat to medium-low. Add remaining $^1/_4$ cup extra-virgin olive oil, yellow onion, and 3 tablespoons garlic, and cook for 5 minutes.

4. Return Jew's mallow leaves to onions. Add 8 cups chicken broth strained to the first pot to onions and Jew's mallow leaves in the second pot. Add remaining 1 teaspoon salt, and cook for 1 hour.

5. Meanwhile, separate chicken meat from bones. Discard bones and remaining contents of first pot.

6. After leaves have been cooking for 1 hour, add chicken, cilantro, cayenne, and remaining 3 tablespoons garlic, and cook for 20 more minutes.

7. Add lemon juice, and cook for 10 more minutes.

8. Serve with brown rice.

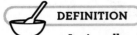 **DEFINITION**

Jew's mallow leaves are leaves of the jute plant and are high in fiber. They're usually sold dried, so to rehydrate the leaves, place them in a large bowl, cover completely with water, and set aside to soak for about 3 hours. Drain, add more water to cover, and soak for 1 more hour.

Okra Stew (*Bamya*)

This stew is a terrific way to change the way okra is served. This stick-to-your-ribs stew marries the distinct flavor of okra with a zesty tomato sauce and tender chunks of chicken.

Yield:	Prep time:	Cook time:	Serving size:
8 cups	20 minutes	40 minutes	1 cup
Each serving has:			
160 calories	8g fat	1g saturated fat	15g protein
8g carbohydrate	3g dietary fiber	32mg cholesterol	639mg sodium

4 TB. extra-virgin olive oil

1 lb. boneless skinless chicken breast, cut into $^1/_2$-in. cubes

4 cups fresh or frozen baby okra

1 large yellow onion, chopped

3 TB. garlic, minced

1 (16-oz.) can plain tomato sauce

2 cups water

1$^1/_2$ tsp. salt

1 tsp. ground black pepper

$^1/_2$ tsp. cayenne

1 cup fresh cilantro, chopped

1. In a 3-quart pot over medium heat, heat 2 tablespoons extra-virgin olive oil. Add chicken, and cook for 5 minutes. Remove chicken to a plate, and set aside.

2. Add remaining 2 tablespoons extra-virgin olive oil to the pot. Add okra and yellow onion, and cook for 7 minutes.

3. Add garlic, and cook for 3 minutes.

4. Return chicken to the pot, and add tomato sauce, water, salt, black pepper, and cayenne. Cook for 20 minutes.

5. Stir in cilantro, and cook for 15 more minutes.

6. Serve warm with brown rice.

Green Pea Stew (*Bazella*)

In this filling stew, warm and soothing green peas are cooked in a tomato sauce with tender carrots and seasoned ground beef.

Yield:	Prep time:	Cook time:	Serving size:
8 cups	15 minutes	43 minutes	1 cup

Each serving has:			
157 calories	9g fat	2g saturated fat	8g protein
12g carbohydrate	1g dietary fiber	17mg cholesterol	628mg sodium

½ lb. ground beef

3 TB. extra-virgin olive oil

1 large yellow onion, finely chopped

2 TB. garlic, minced

2 cups fresh or frozen green peas

2 large carrots, diced (1 cup)

1 (16-oz.) can plain tomato sauce

2 cups water

1½ tsp. salt

1 tsp. ground black pepper

½ cup fresh Italian parsley, finely chopped

1. In a 3-quart pot over medium heat, brown beef for 5 minutes, breaking up chunks with a wooden spoon.

2. Add extra-virgin olive oil, yellow onion, and garlic, and cook for 5 minutes.

3. Add peas and carrots, and cook for 3 minutes.

4. Add tomato sauce, water, salt, and black pepper, and simmer for 25 minutes.

5. Stir in Italian parsley, and simmer for 5 more minutes.

6. Serve warm with brown rice.

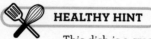 **HEALTHY HINT**

This dish is a great one for kids. It's a good, nutritious way to get little ones to eat some fiber and iron.

Cauliflower Stew

Flavorful cauliflower stew is a great way to incorporate this vegetable into your menu. Tender potatoes and mini meatballs add to the heartiness of this dish.

Yield:	Prep time:	Cook time:	Serving size:
10 cups	20 minutes	25 minutes	2 cups

Each serving has:			
312 calories	6g fat	2g saturated fat	16g protein
50g carbohydrate	9g dietary fiber	27mg cholesterol	1,523mg sodium

¹/₂ lb. ground beef	1 tsp. garlic powder
2 tsp. salt	¹/₂ tsp. onion powder
1 tsp. black pepper	4 cups cauliflower florets
1 (16-oz.) can plain tomato sauce	2 large potatoes
1 (16-oz.) can crushed tomatoes	2 large carrots, finely diced
2 cups water	1 (16-oz.) can chickpeas, rinsed and drained
1 TB. fresh thyme	

1. In a small bowl, combine beef, ¹/₂ teaspoon salt, and ¹/₂ teaspoon black pepper. Form mixture into 20 to 30 mini meatballs about 1 teaspoon each.

2. In a large, 3-quart pot over medium heat, add meatballs. Cover and cook for 5 minutes.

3. Add tomato sauce, crushed tomatoes, water, thyme, garlic powder, onion powder, remaining 1¹/₂ teaspoons salt, and remaining ¹/₂ teaspoon black pepper, and simmer for 5 minutes.

4. Stir in cauliflower, potatoes, carrots, and chickpeas, and simmer for 20 minutes.

5. Serve with brown rice.

Green Bean Stew

Here, green beans pair with tender beef and flavorful tomato sauce.

Yield:	Prep time:	Cook time:	Serving size:
10 cups	50 minutes	$1^1/_2$ hours	1 cup

Each serving has:			
149 calories	7g fat	2g saturated fat	16g protein
6g carbohydrate	1g dietary fiber	26mg cholesterol	756mg sodium

1 lb. beef stew meat, cut into $^1/_2$-in. cubes

1 large yellow onion, chopped

2 bay leaves

6 cups water

2 tsp. salt

3 TB. extra-virgin olive oil

1 lb. green beans, trimmed and cut into 1-in. pieces

3 TB. garlic, minced

1 (16-oz.) can plain tomato sauce

2 TB. tomato paste

2 cups beef broth

1 tsp. ground black pepper

$^1/_2$ tsp. cayenne

1 cup fresh cilantro, chopped

1. In a pressure cooker pot over medium heat, combine beef stew meat, $^1/_2$ of yellow onion, bay leaves, water, and 1 teaspoon salt. Bring to a simmer, and cook, uncovered, for about 10 minutes. Skim off any foam.

2. Add pressure cooker lid, reduce heat to low, and cook for 30 minutes.

3. Release steam from the pressure cooker, and set aside to cool for 30 minutes before removing the lid.

4. In a 3-quart pot over medium heat, heat extra-virgin olive oil. Add green beans and remaining $^1/_2$ of yellow onion, and cook for 7 minutes.

5. Add garlic, and cook for 3 minutes.

6. Return beef to the pot, and add tomato sauce, tomato paste, beef broth, remaining 1 teaspoon salt, black pepper, and cayenne. Cook for 20 minutes.

7. Stir in cilantro, and cook for 15 more minutes.

8. Serve warm with brown rice.

Meaty Mediterranean Lunches

In this chapter, we focus on lunch dishes made with meat—beef, lamb, chicken, and seafood. Many of the recipes call for meat and also a vegetable or grain. It's very rare that you'll find a protein served alone. Remember, the Mediterranean diet is largely a plant-based diet, so the base of most dishes is a vegetable and a grain. This is very important to keep in mind because many of the benefits of the Mediterranean diet come from eating largely plant-based foods.

While the recipes all call for a particular protein, you can easily make substitutions if, for example, you prefer beef to lamb or turkey to chicken. It's a good thing to experiment with recipes and find out what you like.

In This Chapter

- Hearty beef meals
- Tasty lamb lunches
- Flavorful chicken recipes
- Sensational seafood dishes

Beefy Pita Sandwiches

This is a quick, easy, and meaty sandwich with very few ingredients but full of flavor.

Yield:	Prep time:	Cook time:	Serving size:
4 pita sandwiches	10 minutes	20 minutes	1 pita sandwich

Each serving has:			
409 calories	19g fat	6g saturated fat	25g protein
33g carbohydrate	2g dietary fiber	66mg cholesterol	884mg sodium

1 lb. ground beef	1 tsp. seven spices
1 tsp. salt	4 (6- or 7-in.) pitas
¹/₂ tsp. ground black pepper	

1. Preheat the oven to 400°F.

2. In a medium bowl, combine beef, salt, black pepper, and seven spices.

3. Lay out pitas on the counter, and divide beef mixture evenly among them, and spread beef to edge of pitas.

4. Place pitas on a baking sheet, and bake for 20 minutes.

5. Serve warm with Greek yogurt.

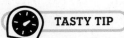 **TASTY TIP**

For a little more kick, you can add a finely chopped jalapeño pepper. It adds great flavor and spice.

Kefta Burgers

This recipe turns the American burger into a Mediterranean burger! The juicy, seasoned burger is served with a tahini mayonnaise on a fresh mini pita.

Yield:	Prep time:	Cook time:	Serving size:
4 burgers	20 minutes	10 minutes	1 burger

Each serving has:			
613 calories	35g fat	8g saturated fat	28g protein
48g carbohydrate	4g dietary fiber	74g cholesterol	1,400mg sodium

1 lb. ground beef	1/2 cup mayonnaise
1 cup fresh parsley, finely chopped	3 TB. tahini paste
1 tsp. seven spices	2 TB. balsamic vinegar
1 1/2 tsp. salt	1/2 tsp. ground black pepper
1 large yellow onion, finely sliced	4 (4-in.) pitas
1 TB. sumac	1 medium tomato, sliced

1. In a large bowl, combine beef, 1/2 cup parsley, seven spices, 1 teaspoon salt. Form mixture into 4 patties.

2. In a medium bowl, combine remaining 1/2 cup parsley, yellow onion, and sumac.

3. In a small bowl, whisk together mayonnaise, tahini paste, remaining 1/2 teaspoon salt, balsamic vinegar, and black pepper.

4. Preheat a large skillet over medium-high heat. Place patties in the skillet, and cook for 5 minutes per side.

5. To assemble burgers, open each pita into a pocket, and spread both sides with tahini mayonnaise. Add 1 burger patty, some parsley mixture, and a few tomato slices, and serve.

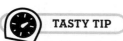 **TASTY TIP**

If you don't have pitas, a good alternative is a toasted English muffin.

Baked Spaghetti with Beef

Baked spaghetti was my mom's go-to dish when we came home from school and wanted something fun to eat. Tender noodles with bits of browned beef and a herb seasoned sauce—kids of any age will love it.

Yield:	Prep time:	Cook time:	Serving size:
10 cups	20 minutes	$1^1/_2$ hours	1 cup

Each serving has:			
368 calories	13g fat	4g saturated fat	18g protein
44g carbohydrate	3g dietary fiber	34mg cholesterol	972mg sodium

1 lb. ground beef

1 large yellow onion, finely chopped

$^1/_2$ medium green bell pepper, ribs and seeds removed, and finely chopped

2 TB. minced garlic

4 TB. extra-virgin olive oil

2 (16-oz.) can plain tomato sauce

1 (16-oz.) can diced tomatoes, with juice

3 TB. tomato paste

2 cups water

2 TB. sugar

$2^1/_2$ tsp. salt

1 tsp. dried oregano

1 tsp. dried thyme

$^1/_3$ cup fresh basil, chopped

3 TB. fresh Italian parsley, chopped

$^1/_2$ tsp. crushed red pepper flakes

$^1/_2$ tsp. ground black pepper

1 lb. spaghetti

1 cup shredded mozzarella cheese

1. In a large, 3-quart pot over medium heat, brown beef for 5 minutes, breaking up chunks with a wooden spoon.

2. Stir in yellow onion, green bell pepper, garlic, and extra-virgin olive oil, and cook for 5 minutes.

3. Add tomato sauce, diced tomatoes with juice, tomato paste, water, sugar, $1^1/_2$ teaspoons salt, oregano, thyme, basil, Italian parsley, crushed red pepper flakes, and black pepper, and stir. Reduce heat to low, and cook for 20 minutes.

4. Bring another large pot of water to a boil over high heat. Add remaining 1 teaspoon salt and spaghetti, and boil for 8 minutes.

5. Preheat the oven to 450°F.

6. Drain spaghetti, and pour into a large casserole dish. Add pasta sauce, and toss to combine. Cover with a piece of aluminum foil, and bake for 20 minutes.

7. Remove the casserole dish from the oven, remove the foil, and evenly sprinkle mozzarella cheese over spaghetti. Return the casserole dish to the oven, and bake for 15 more minutes.

8. Let spaghetti rest for 10 minutes before serving.

Hearty Meat and Potatoes

Tender meat and potatoes take on new flavors with sweet sautéed onions and warm seven spices.

Yield:	Prep time:	Cook time:	Serving size:
8 cups	10 minutes	30 minutes	2 cups
Each serving has:			
662 calories	27g fat	7g saturated fat	28g protein
77g carbohydrate	12g dietary fiber	66mg cholesterol	971mg sodium

1 lb. ground beef or lamb	1¹/₂ tsp. salt
¹/₄ cup extra-virgin olive oil	1 TB. seven spices
1 large yellow onion, chopped	¹/₂ tsp. ground black pepper
5 large potatoes, peeled and cubed	

1. In a large, 3-quart pot over medium heat, brown beef for 5 minutes, breaking up chunks with a wooden spoon.

2. Add extra-virgin olive oil and yellow onion, and cook for 5 minutes.

3. Toss in potatoes, salt, seven spices, and black pepper. Cover and cook for 10 minutes. Toss gently, and cook for 10 more minutes.

4. Serve warm with a side of Greek yogurt.

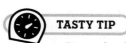 **TASTY TIP**

Be gentle when tossing the potatoes—you don't want them to turn to mush. Try using a metal spoon to gently toss them in the pan.

Beef-Stuffed Squash (*Kusa Mihshi*)

I love this dish because it's so easy to make and you really don't need any sides with it. The zucchini squash is filled with a seasoned rice and meat mixture and cooked in a flavorful tomato sauce.

Yield:	Prep time:	Cook time:	Serving size:
8 zucchini	30 minutes	1 hour	1 zucchini

Each serving has:			
180 calories	7g fat	3g saturated fat	14g protein
17g carbohydrate	3g dietary fiber	33mg cholesterol	1,268mg sodium

8 (5-in.) light green zucchini	1 tsp. ground black pepper
1 cup long-grain rice, rinsed	4 cups plain tomato sauce
1 lb. ground beef	2 cups water
2 TB. minced garlic	1 tsp. dried mint
2 tsp. salt	

1. Trim off top of zucchini, and using a zucchini corer or a teaspoon, core zucchini. Set aside.

2. In a large bowl, combine long-grain rice, beef, 1 tablespoon garlic, 1 teaspoon salt, and $^1/_2$ teaspoon black pepper.

3. Loosely stuff each zucchini with 3 or 4 tablespoons rice mixture. Do not overstuff.

4. In a large pot over low heat, combine tomato sauce, water, remaining 1 tablespoon garlic, remaining 1 teaspoon salt, remaining $^1/_2$ teaspoon black pepper, and mint.

5. Add stuffed zucchini to tomato sauce, cover, and cook for 1 hour.

6. Serve warm.

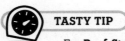 **TASTY TIP**

For **Beef-Stuffed Squash in Garlic Yogurt Sauce,** replace the tomato sauce with 4 cups plain Greek yogurt.

Beef-Stuffed Baked Potatoes

Here, tender potatoes are stuffed with a seasoned meat filling and baked in an earthy tomato sauce. This filling dish is a good source of fiber and protein.

Yield:	Prep time:	Cook time:	Serving size:
6 potatoes	30 minutes	25 minutes	1 potato

Each serving has:			
525 calories	19g fat	5g saturated fat	21g protein
69g carbohydrate	8g dietary fiber	44mg cholesterol	1,058mg sodium

1 lb. ground beef	1 (16-oz.) can plain tomato sauce
1 large white onion, finely chopped	1 TB. fresh thyme
4 TB. extra-virgin olive oil	1 tsp. dried oregano
1 TB. seven spices	1 tsp. ground black pepper
2 tsp. salt	$^1/_2$ tsp. garlic powder
6 large potatoes, peeled	

1. In a large skillet over medium heat, brown beef for 5 minutes, breaking up chunks with a wooden spoon.

2. Add white onion, 2 tablespoons extra-virgin olive oil, seven spices, and 1 teaspoon salt, and cook for 5 minutes.

3. Preheat the oven to 450°F.

4. Trim bottoms of potatoes so they'll stand on end. Cut off the top $^1/_4$ of potatoes, and set aside. Core out inside of potatoes and set aside to use in another recipe.

5. Stand potatoes inside a large casserole dish. Fill each potato with 3 tablespoons meat mixture, and place potato tops back on potatoes. Evenly drizzle potatoes with remaining 2 tablespoons extra-virgin olive oil, and bake for 15 minutes.

6. Meanwhile, in a 2-quart pot over medium heat, combine tomato sauce, remaining 1 teaspoon salt, thyme, oregano, black pepper, and garlic powder. Simmer for 10 minutes.

7. After potatoes have baked for 15 minutes, pour sauce mixture in the casserole dish around potatoes, and bake for 10 minutes.

8. Serve warm.

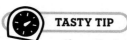 **TASTY TIP**

If you don't want beef, you can replace it with lamb or even ground turkey instead.

Lamb-Stuffed Baked Peppers

If you like bell peppers, you'll love this dish because they're the main attraction, filled with seasoned rice and ground lamb and topped with a zesty tomato sauce.

Yield:	Prep time:	Cook time:	Serving size:
4 peppers	40 minutes	$1^{1}/_{2}$ hours	1 pepper

Each serving has:			
447 calories	24g fat	7g saturated fat	25g protein
33g carbohydrate	6g dietary fiber	66mg cholesterol	1,865mg sodium

1 lb. ground lamb or beef	1 tsp. ground black pepper
1 medium yellow onion, chopped	1 tsp. turmeric
2 TB. minced garlic	1 cup long-grain rice
3 TB. extra-virgin olive oil	3 cups water
1 large tomato, chopped	1 (16-oz.) can plain tomato sauce
1 large carrot, shredded	1 TB. sugar
$^{1}/_{4}$ cup plus 2 TB. fresh basil, chopped	4 large green, red, yellow, or orange sweet bell peppers
$2^{1}/_{2}$ tsp. salt	

1. In a large skillet over medium heat, brown lamb for 5 minutes, breaking up chunks with a wooden spoon.

2. Add yellow onion, garlic, extra-virgin olive oil, tomato, carrot, $^{1}/_{4}$ cup basil, $1^{1}/_{2}$ teaspoons salt, black pepper, and turmeric, and cook for 7 minutes.

3. Add long-grain rice and 2 cups water to the skillet, cover, and cook for 30 minutes. Remove from heat.

4. In a 2-quart pot over medium heat, combine tomato sauce, remaining 1 teaspoon salt, remaining 2 tablespoons basil, remaining 1 cup water, and sugar. Stir and simmer for 10 minutes.

5. Preheat the oven to 450°F.

6. Cut off tops of green bell peppers, and remove ribs and seeds. Stand peppers in a 8×8-inch casserole dish (if they won't stand, trim them slightly so they will), and fill each with about 1 cup rice mixture.

7. Bake for 15 minutes. Remove the casserole dish from the oven, and reduce the temperature to 400°F.

8. Spoon tomato sauce over each bell pepper and into the casserole dish. Add pepper tops to peppers, cover the casserole dish with aluminum foil, bake for 20 minutes.

9. Let peppers rest for 10 minutes before serving.

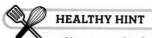 **HEALTHY HINT**

You can make this recipe healthier by using brown rice instead of long-grain rice. The brown rice adds a more earthy taste and texture.

Lamb Cabbage Rolls (*Malfouf*)

In this hearty dish, cabbage leaves are stuffed with a seasoned lamb and rice mixture and cooked in a mild garlic tomato sauce.

Yield:	Prep time:	Cook time:	Serving size:
24 rolls	40 minutes	1^1/$_2$ hours	2 rolls
Each serving has:			
141 calories	5g fat	2g saturated fat	9g protein
15g carbohydrate	4g dietary fiber	25mg cholesterol	856mg sodium

1 large head green cabbage	1 tsp. ground black pepper
1 cup long-grain rice, rinsed	4 cups plain tomato sauce
1 lb. ground lamb	2 cups water
4 TB. minced garlic	1 tsp. dried mint
2 tsp. salt	

1. Using a knife, cut around core of cabbage and remove core. Place head of cabbage, core side down, in a large pot. Cover with water, and cook over high heat for 30 minutes. Drain, cool cabbage, and separate leaves. You need 24 leaves.

2. In a large bowl, combine long-grain rice, lamb, 1 tablespoon minced garlic, 1 teaspoon salt, and ^{1}/$_2$ teaspoon black pepper.

3. In a 2-quart pot, combine tomato sauce, water, remaining 3 tablespoons garlic, mint, remaining 1 teaspoon salt, and remaining ^{1}/$_2$ teaspoon black pepper.

4. Lay each cabbage leaf flat, spoon 2 tablespoons filling on each leaf, and roll. Layer rolls in a large pot, pour sauce into the pot, cover, and cook over medium-low heat for 1 hour.

5. Let rolls rest for 20 minutes before serving warm with Greek yogurt.

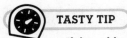 **TASTY TIP**

If the cabbage leaves are too large, you can cut them in half when making these cabbage rolls.

Cheeseless Meat Pizza (*Lahme bi Ajeen*)

You'll love this pizza. Tender, flaky dough is topped with minced meat mixed with zesty spices, tomatoes, and onions. Who needs cheese or sauce?

Yield:	Prep time:	Cook time:	Serving size:
6 pizzas	3 hours	20 minutes	1 pizza

Each serving has:			
619 calories	24g fat	7g saturated fat	30g protein
69g carbohydrate	4g dietary fiber	70mg cholesterol	849mg sodium

1 batch Multipurpose Dough (recipe in Chapter 12)	1 TB. seven spices
1 lb. ground beef	1 tsp. salt
1/2 lb. ground lamb	1/2 tsp. ground black pepper
1 large tomato, finely diced	1/2 cup cornmeal
1 large yellow onion, finely chopped	

1. Preheat the oven to 450°F. Sprinkle a baking sheet with some cornmeal.

2. Cut Multipurpose Dough into 6 equal portions, and roll each into a 7-inch circle.

3. In a medium bowl, combine beef, lamb, tomato, yellow onion, seven spices, salt, and black pepper. Divide mixture into 6 equal portions, place 1 on top of each rolled-out dough circle, and spread meat mixture evenly over dough.

4. Place pizzas on the prepared baking sheet, but do not overcrowd. Bake for 20 minutes.

5. Serve warm with a side of Greek yogurt.

Breaded Chicken (Chicken *Escalope*)

Breaded chicken doesn't have to be deep-fried! This version is pan-fried with a little bit of olive oil and has a well-seasoned, crispy crust on the outside while remaining moist and tender on the inside.

Yield:	Prep time:	Cook time:	Serving size:
8 pieces	15 minutes	12 minutes	1 (2-ounce) piece

Each serving has:			
388 calories	18g fat	3g saturated fat	21g protein
36g carbohydrate	3g dietary fiber	63mg cholesterol	1,172mg sodium

2 (8-oz.) boneless, skinless chicken breasts	2 cups panko breadcrumbs or crushed cornflakes cereal
2 tsp. salt	1 TB. dried thyme
1^1/$_2$ tsp. ground black pepper	1 TB. dried oregano
1 cup whole milk	1 TB. dried marjoram
1 large egg	1 TB. paprika
1 cup all-purpose flour	^{1}/$_2$ cup extra-virgin olive oil

1. Cut chicken breasts in half, holding the knife horizontally so you yield 2 thin pieces. Then cut each piece in half along the width for a total of 8 pieces. Evenly season chicken with 1 teaspoon salt and ^{1}/$_2$ teaspoon black pepper.

2. In a shallow bowl, whisk together whole milk and egg. Set aside.

3. Place all-purpose flour in another shallow bowl and panko breadcrumbs in a third shallow bowl. To each bowl add ^{1}/$_2$ teaspoon salt, ^{1}/$_2$ teaspoon black pepper, ^{1}/$_2$ tablespoon thyme, ^{1}/$_2$ tablespoon oregano, ^{1}/$_2$ tablespoon marjoram, and ^{1}/$_2$ tablespoon paprika, and stir to combine.

4. Arrange the bowls in an assembly-line fashion. Drench chicken in seasoned flour, coat in milk-and-egg mixture, coat with seasoned breadcrumbs, and set on a plate. Repeat with remaining chicken pieces.

5. Preheat a skillet over medium heat, add extra-virgin olive oil, and heat for about 2 minutes. Add chicken to the skillet, but do not overcrowd the skillet. Cook chicken for 5 minutes per side.

6. Serve warm.

Chicken Phyllo Rolls (*Msakhan*)

These flaky phyllo rolls are filled with tangy seasoned chicken and sweet onions. They're perfect as finger food or a light lunch.

Yield:	Prep time:	Cook time:	Serving size:
12 rolls	20 minutes	35 minutes	1 roll
Each serving has:			
356 calories	25g fat	12g saturated fat	12g protein
21g carbohydrate	1g dietary fiber	81mg cholesterol	514mg sodium

3 TB. extra-virgin olive oil	2 TB. sumac
1 lb. ground chicken	1 pkg. frozen phyllo dough (12 sheets)
1 large white onion, finely chopped	
1 tsp. salt	1 cup butter, melted

1. In a large skillet over medium heat, heat extra-virgin olive oil. Add chicken, and brown for 5 minutes, breaking up chunks with a wooden spoon.

2. Add white onion and salt, and cook for 5 minutes.

3. Remove the skillet from heat, stir in sumac, and set aside to cool.

4. Preheat the oven to 450°F.

5. Lay first sheet of phyllo on a plate, brush with melted butter. Place second sheet of phyllo on top, and brush with melted butter. Cut sheets in half.

6. Place 3 tablespoons chicken mixture at end of phyllo, fold over sides, and roll phyllo with filling. Place on a baking sheet, and brush top with more melted butter. Bake for 15 minutes or until golden brown.

7. Serve warm.

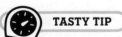 **TASTY TIP**

You can make a large number of these rolls and freeze them for quick, grab-and-go lunches later. After rolling the phyllo dough and adding the filling, place the rolls on a baking sheet and freeze. When they're frozen, transfer the rolls to a plastic bag.

Chicken Quinoa Pilaf

Quinoa is an amazing superfood. This nutty-tasting seed contains lots of protein and fiber. This dish combines quinoa's earthy flavor with sweet tomatoes, juicy chicken, and pungent olives.

Yield:	Prep time:	Cook time:	Serving size:
8 cups	20 minutes	35 minutes	1 cup

Each serving has:			
183 calories	7g fat	1g saturated fat	16g protein
14g carbohydrate	3g dietary fiber	32mg cholesterol	658mg sodium

2 (8-oz.) boneless, skinless chicken breasts, cut into $^1/_2$-in. cubes

3 TB. extra-virgin olive oil

1 medium red onion, finely chopped

1 TB. minced garlic

1 (16-oz.) can diced tomatoes, with juice

2 cups water

2 tsp. salt

1 TB. dried oregano

1 TB. turmeric

1 tsp. paprika

1 tsp. ground black pepper

2 cups red or yellow quinoa

$^1/_2$ cup fresh parsley, chopped

1. In a large, 3-quart pot over medium heat, heat extra-virgin olive oil. Add chicken, and cook for 5 minutes.

2. Add red onion and garlic, stir, and cook for 5 minutes.

3. Add tomatoes with juice, water, salt, oregano, turmeric, paprika, and black pepper. Stir, and simmer for 5 minutes.

4. Add red quinoa, and stir. Cover, reduce heat to low, and cook for 20 minutes. Remove from heat.

5. Fluff with a fork, cover again, and let sit for 10 minutes.

6. Serve warm.

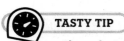 **TASTY TIP**

If you don't like oregano or parsley, you can easily replace them with any herb you like.

Fish with Tahini Sauce (Fish Tagine)

This fish dish is full of bright flavors. The light and flaky fish is baked in a tangy tahini sauce and topped with sweet, sautéed onions and toasted pine nuts.

Yield:	Prep time:	Cook time:	Serving size:
4 fillets	20 minutes	41 minutes	1 fillet

Each serving has:			
892 calories	65g fat	13g saturated fat	69g protein
17g carbohydrate	6g dietary fiber	161mg cholesterol	1,406mg sodium

4 (8-oz.) tilapia fillets	1 cup water
2 tsp. salt	1 TB. minced garlic
1 tsp. ground black pepper	1 TB. dried cilantro
3 TB. plus 1 tsp. extra-virgin olive oil	$^{1}/_{2}$ tsp. cayenne
$^{3}/_{4}$ cup tahini paste	4 TB. butter
$^{1}/_{3}$ cup lemon juice	2 large yellow onions, sliced
$^{1}/_{3}$ cup Greek yogurt	$^{1}/_{2}$ cup pine nuts

1. Preheat the oven to 450°F.

2. Season both sides of tilapia with $^{1}/_{2}$ teaspoon salt and black pepper.

3. In a nonstick pan over high heat, heat 3 tablespoons extra-virgin olive oil. Add tilapia, and cook for 2 minutes per side. Transfer tilapia to a casserole dish.

4. In a large bowl, combine tahini paste, lemon juice, Greek yogurt, water, garlic, cilantro, cayenne, and 1 teaspoon salt. Pour tahini sauce over tilapia, and bake for 15 minutes.

5. Meanwhile, in a large skillet over medium-low heat, heat butter. Add yellow onions and remaining $^{1}/_{2}$ teaspoon salt, and cook for 20 minutes or until onions are golden and caramelized. Remove from heat.

6. In a small saucepan over medium-low heat, heat remaining 1 teaspoon extra-virgin olive oil. Add pine nuts, and toast for 2 minutes or until golden brown. Remove from heat.

7. To serve, spoon caramelized onions over tilapia and tahini sauce, and sprinkle toasted pine nuts over top. Serve with pita bread or pita chips.

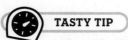 **TASTY TIP**

If you like the flavor of cilantro, you can sprinkle some fresh chopped cilantro on top before serving.

Lemon Cilantro Shrimp

I love shrimp with a lot of flavor, and this dish certainly has flavor, thanks to the zesty lemon, fresh herbs, and a little punch of garlic.

Yield:	Prep time:	Cook time:	Serving size:
5 cups	10 minutes	5 minutes	1 cup

Each serving has:			
176 calories	10g fat	1g saturated fat	19g protein
3g carbohydrate	0g dietary fiber	138mg cholesterol	368mg sodium

3 TB. extra-virgin olive oil	$^1/_2$ tsp. ground black pepper
2 TB. minced garlic	$^1/_2$ tsp. cayenne
1 lb. fresh medium shrimp (about 36 to 40), shells and veins removed	$^1/_4$ cup fresh lemon juice
	$^1/_2$ cup fresh cilantro, chopped
$^1/_2$ tsp. salt	

1. In a large skillet over medium heat, heat extra-virgin olive oil. Add garlic, and cook for 1 minute.

2. Add shrimp, salt, black pepper, and cayenne; toss; and cook for 3 minutes.

3. Add lemon juice and cilantro, toss, and cook for 1 more minute.

4. Serve warm.

 MEDITERRANEAN MORSEL

The worst thing you can do to shrimp is overcook it; they become rubbery and hard to chew. Remember, when you remove the shrimp from the heat, they continue to cook, so don't overcook them while they're in the pan.

Grilled Shrimp Sandwiches with Pesto

This sandwich features the robust flavors of pesto and Havarti cheese with mildly seasoned shrimp and peppery arugula.

Yield:	Prep time:	Cook time:	Serving size:
5 sandwiches	20 minutes	4 minutes	1 sandwich

Each serving has:			
646 calories	45g fat	11g saturated fat	35g protein
27g carbohydrate	3g dietary fiber	209mg cholesterol	1,168mg sodium

1 lb. fresh medium shrimp (36 to 40), shells and veins removed

1 tsp. salt

$1^1/_2$ tsp. ground black pepper

$^1/_3$ cup plus 4 TB. extra-virgin olive oil

4 cups fresh basil leaves

3 large cloves garlic

$^1/_4$ cup lemon juice

$^1/_3$ cup toasted pine nuts

$^1/_3$ cup grated Parmesan cheese

3 cups fresh arugula

3 TB. balsamic vinegar

5 slices Havarti cheese

5 panini rolls, split

1. Preheat a grill to medium heat.

2. In a medium bowl, toss shrimp with $^1/_2$ teaspoon salt, $^1/_2$ teaspoon black pepper, and 2 tablespoons extra-virgin olive oil. Thread shrimp onto skewers, and grill for 2 minutes per side. Set aside.

3. In a food processor fitted with a chopping blade, blend basil, remaining $^1/_2$ teaspoon salt, $^1/_2$ teaspoon black pepper, garlic, lemon juice, pine nuts, Parmesan cheese, and $^1/_3$ cup extra-virgin olive oil for 2 minutes, intermittently scraping down the sides of the food processor bowl with a rubber spatula.

4. In a small bowl, toss arugula with remaining 2 tablespoons extra-virgin olive oil, balsamic vinegar, and remaining $^1/_2$ teaspoon black pepper.

5. To assemble sandwiches, spread 1 tablespoon pesto on each side of rolls, add $^1/_5$ of shrimp, 1 slice Havarti cheese, $^1/_5$ of arugula, and other half of rolls. Serve immediately.

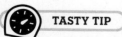 **TASTY TIP**

Toasting your bread adds a lot of flavor to a sandwich. Try toasting your bread on the grill or in a toaster before assembling the sandwich.

Shrimp and Vegetable Rice

With tender, perfectly cooked shrimp and seasoned brown rice, this dish is filling and healthy.

Yield:	Prep time:	Cook time:	Serving size:
8 cups	20 minutes	48 minutes	1 cup

Each serving has:			
27 calories	7g fat	1g saturated fat	11g protein
42g carbohydrate	3g dietary fiber	55mg cholesterol	658mg sodium

3 TB. extra-virgin olive oil

1 medium yellow onion, finely chopped

1 TB. minced garlic

1 cup green peas

2 medium carrots, shredded (1 cup)

4 cups water

2 tsp. salt

10 strands saffron

1 tsp. turmeric

$^1/_2$ tsp. black pepper

2 cups brown rice

$^1/_2$ lb. medium raw shrimp (18 to 20), shells and veins removed

1. In a large, 3-quart pot over medium heat, heat extra-virgin olive oil. Add yellow onion, and cook for 5 minutes.

2. Add garlic, green peas, and carrots, and cook for 3 minutes.

3. Add water, salt, saffron, turmeric, and black pepper; bring to a boil; and cook for about 3 minutes.

4. Add brown rice, cover, reduce heat to low, and cook for 30 minutes.

5. Gently fold shrimp into rice, cover, and cook for 10 minutes.

6. Remove from heat, fluff with a fork, cover, and set aside for 10 minutes. Serve warm.

Basil and Shrimp Quinoa

This tasty dish combines the earthy flavor of quinoa with fresh herbs and tender shrimp.

Yield:	Prep time:	Cook time:	Serving size:
8 cups	20 minutes	20 minutes	1 cup

Each serving has:			
160 calories	7g fat	1g saturated fat	11g protein
14g carbohydrate	2g dietary fiber	55mg cholesterol	543mg sodium

3 TB. extra-virgin olive oil

2 TB. minced garlic

1 cup fresh broccoli florets

3 stalks asparagus, chopped (1 cup)

4 cups chicken or vegetable broth

1¹/₂ tsp. salt

1 tsp. ground black pepper

1 TB. lemon zest

2 cups red quinoa

¹/₂ cup fresh basil, chopped

¹/₂ lb. medium raw shrimp (18 to 20), shells and veins removed

1. In a 2-quart pot over low heat, heat extra-virgin olive oil. Add garlic, and cook for 3 minutes.

2. Increase heat to medium, add broccoli and asparagus, and cook for 2 minutes.

3. Add chicken broth, salt, black pepper, and lemon zest, and bring to a boil. Stir in red quinoa, cover, and cook for 15 minutes.

4. Fold in basil and shrimp, cover, and cook for 10 minutes.

5. Remove from heat, fluff with a fork, cover, and set aside for 10 minutes. Serve warm.

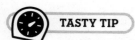 **TASTY TIP**

If you like ginger, you can add 1 tablespoon finely chopped ginger when you add the broccoli and asparagus for a very refreshing flavor.

Very Vegetarian Lunches

Many people think vegetarian meals aren't as filling as dishes that contain meat, but the recipes in this chapter prove that notion wrong! The vegetarian dishes in this chapter are just as satisfying as any dish containing meat.

Even if you're not a vegetarian, it's still a good idea to introduce a few meatless meals into your menu from time to time to give your body a break from meat. You'll also reap more benefits of more vegetables in your diet.

The key is to serve the dish with a whole grain like brown rice, pilaf, or whole-wheat pasta to keep you full longer. For example, Eggplant Casserole (*Moussaka*) would go great with Bulgur Chickpea Pilaf (recipe in Chapter 10).

In This Chapter

- Filling vegetarian lunches
- Flavorful Mediterranean dishes
- Hearty casserole and grains
- Sensational sandwiches

Falafel Pita Pockets

Falafel are flavorful, golf ball–size, fried patties made of hearty beans, fresh herbs, and zesty spices. They go great in a sandwich or on their own with a tangy tahini dipping sauce.

Yield:	Prep time:	Cook time:	Serving size:
8 pita pockets	9^1/$_2$ hours	10 minutes	1 pita pocket

Each serving has:			
246 calories	15g fat	2g saturated fat	8g protein
24g carbohydrate	6g dietary fiber	0mg cholesterol	581mg sodium

1^1/$_2$ cups dried chickpeas

1^1/$_2$ cups dried fava beans

6 cups water

1 cup fresh cilantro, chopped

^{1}/$_2$ cup fresh parsley, chopped

1 large yellow onion, roughly chopped

6 cloves garlic

3 tsp. salt

2 TB. ground coriander seeds

1 TB. ground cumin

1 tsp. ground black pepper

^{1}/$_2$ tsp. cayenne

^{1}/$_4$ cup plain breadcrumbs

3 TB. all-purpose flour

1 TB. baking soda

1 TB. baking powder

8 cups vegetable oil

4 (6-in.) pitas

2 large tomatoes, sliced

Pickled Turnips (*Kabees;* recipe in Chapter 18)

2 cups shredded lettuce

Tahini Sauce (*Tarator;* recipe in Chapter 13)

1. In a large bowl, combine chickpeas and fava beans with water. Set aside to soak overnight or for 8 or 9 hours.

2. Drain beans, and add them to a food processor fitted with a chopping blade. Blend for 2 minutes, intermittently stopping to scrape down the sides of the bowl with a rubber spatula. Transfer bean mixture back to the large bowl.

3. In the food processor, blend cilantro, parsley, yellow onion, garlic, salt, coriander, cumin, black pepper, and cayenne for 1 minute or until smooth. Transfer mixture to the large bowl.

4. Add breadcrumbs, all-purpose flour, baking soda, and baking powder to the bowl, and mix well. Set aside for 15 minutes.

5. In a large pot over medium heat, heat vegetable oil to 365°F. Using an ice-cream scoop or 2 spoons, form falafel mixture into golf ball–size patties. Carefully drop falafel balls in oil, and fry for about 4 minutes or until dark golden brown. Do not overcrowd the pot.

6. Remove falafel from oil, and transfer to a plate lined with paper towels to drain.

7. To assemble, cut pitas in half and open the pockets. Place 3 falafel balls in the pocket, and add some tomatoes, Pickled Turnips (*Kabees*), and lettuce. Drizzle with Tahini Sauce (*Tarator*), and serve.

 HEALTHY HINT

Falafel is a staple in the Mediterranean region. Aside from the fact that it is fried, it is full of fiber, protein, and antioxidants. You can make it a bit healthier by frying it in a light olive oil—or even baking it. Why use dried chickpeas and fava beans and then rehydrate them instead of using canned? Canned chickpeas and beans are cooked, so they have a different texture. Rehydrated chickpeas and beans are uncooked; they're just rehydrated and, therefore, have a firmer texture. If you use canned beans, the texture will be mushy and will disintegrate when you try to fry the balls.

Couscous with Vegetable Stew

Couscous can be prepared many different ways. Pairing fluffy couscous topped with a warm and flavorful vegetable stew is ideal on any cold day.

Yield:	Prep time:	Cook time:	Serving size:
8 cups	30 minutes	27 minutes	1 cup

Each serving has:			
210 calories	6g fat	1g saturated fat	6g protein
35g carbohydrate	6g dietary fiber	0mg cholesterol	1,281mg sodium

3 TB. extra-virgin olive oil

1 large yellow onion, finely chopped

2 medium zucchini, cut into cubes

3 large carrots, peeled and sliced

1 TB. minced garlic

4 cups plain tomato sauce

5 cups water

$1^1/_2$ tsp. salt

1 tsp. seven spices

1 tsp. paprika

$^1/_2$ tsp. cayenne

$^1/_2$ tsp. ground nutmeg

1 tsp. fresh thyme

1 (16-oz.) can chickpeas, drained

1 large potato, peeled and cut into cubes

$^1/_4$ cup fresh parsley, finely chopped

$^1/_4$ cup fresh cilantro, finely chopped

1 vegetable bouillon cube

2 cups instant couscous

1. In a large pot over medium heat, heat extra-virgin olive oil. Add yellow onion, and cook for 5 minutes.

2. Add zucchini, carrots, and garlic, and cook for 5 minutes.

3. Add tomato sauce, 2 cups water, salt, seven spices, paprika, cayenne, nutmeg, thyme, and chickpeas, and gently stir. Reduce heat to low, and cook for 10 minutes.

4. Stir in potato, parsley, and cilantro, and cook for 5 minutes. Remove from heat.

5. In medium saucepan over medium heat, bring 3 cups water and vegetable bouillon to a simmer. Add couscous, and cook for 2 minutes. Remove from heat, cover and set aside for 10 minutes. Fluff couscous with a fork, cover, and set aside for 5 more minutes.

6. To serve, spoon couscous onto a plate and top with 1 cup stew on top.

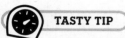 **TASTY TIP**

Couscous is a lot like pasta; it's a blank pallet that needs to be colored with flavor. Try pairing couscous with different sauces and stews and finding new favorite combinations.

Sweet and Savory Couscous

Here, sweet raisins combine with fluffy couscous that's seasoned with spices and herbs. The added vegetables make it flavorful and filling.

Yield:	Prep time:	Cook time:	Serving size:
5 cups	20 minutes	23 minutes	1 cup
Each serving has:			
458 calories	21g fat	3g saturated fat	19g protein
53g carbohydrate	5g dietary fiber	3mg cholesterol	2,068mg sodium

3 TB. extra-virgin olive oil	$^1/_2$ tsp. ground cloves
1 large white onion, finely chopped	$^1/_2$ tsp. ground cinnamon
$^1/_2$ cup pine nuts	$^1/_2$ tsp. ground allspice
2 large carrots, chopped	$^1/_2$ tsp. ground ginger
1 cup green peas	1 tsp. seven spices
1 cup golden raisins	1 tsp. ground coriander seeds
5 cups vegetable broth	$^1/_4$ cup fresh parsley, finely chopped
1 tsp. salt	2 cups instant couscous

1. In a large pot over medium heat, heat extra-virgin olive oil. Add white onion, and cook, stirring with a wooden spoon, for 5 minutes.

2. Add pine nuts, and cook for 3 more minutes.

3. Add carrots, green peas, and golden raisins, and cook for 3 minutes.

4. Add vegetable broth, salt, cloves, cinnamon, allspice, ginger, seven spices, and coriander, and cook for 10 minutes.

5. Add parsley and couscous, and cook for 2 minutes. Remove from heat, cover, and set aside for 10 minutes. Fluff couscous with a fork, cover, and set aside for 5 more minutes. Serve warm.

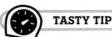   **TASTY TIP**

When you want to reheat the couscous, add 2 or 3 tablespoons water to it before reheating. This gives it some moisture and helps keep it from clumping.

Macaroni with Yogurt Sauce

In this light and refreshing dish, elbow macaroni combine with a smooth and creamy yogurt sauce, a hint of fresh mint, and a crunch from toasted pine nuts.

Yield:	Prep time:	Cook time:	Serving size:
6 cups	10 minutes	10 minutes	1 cup
Each serving has:			
259 calories	13g fat	1g saturated fat	16g protein
20g carbohydrate	1g dietary fiber	6mg cholesterol	624mg sodium

6 cups water	1 tsp. dried mint
$1^{1}/_{2}$ tsp. salt	1 tsp. minced garlic
$^{1}/_{2}$ lb. elbow macaroni	$^{1}/_{2}$ tsp. ground black pepper
3 cups plain Greek yogurt	2 TB. extra-virgin olive oil
3 TB. fresh mint, chopped	$^{1}/_{2}$ cup pine nuts

1. In a large, 3-quart pot over high heat, bring water and $^{1}/_{2}$ teaspoon salt to a boil. Add elbow macaroni, and cook for 8 minutes. Drain.

2. In a large bowl, whisk together Greek yogurt, fresh mint, dried mint, garlic, remaining 1 teaspoon salt, and black pepper. Add cooked pasta, and mix well.

3. In a small saucepan over low heat, heat extra-virgin olive oil. Add pine nuts, and toast for 2 minutes.

4. Spoon toasted pine nuts over yogurt and pasta, and serve warm or cold.

MEDITERRANEAN MORSEL

If you like meat with your pasta, you could add some browned ground beef atop this dish for another layer of flavor and protein.

Vegetable Grape Leaves

I love veggie grape leaves because you can eat them any time of day. Here, the zesty rice and vegetable filling is rolled in a tender grape leaf and cooked in a citrus broth.

Yield:	Prep time:	Cook time:	Serving size:
4 dozen	1 hour, 15 minutes	$1^1/_2$ hours	2 rolls

Each serving has:			
100 calories	8g fat	1g saturated fat	1g protein
8g carbohydrate	1g dietary fiber	0mg cholesterol	735mg sodium

2 cups long-grain rice, rinsed

1 cup fresh parsley, finely chopped

1 large tomato, finely diced

1 medium yellow onion, finely chopped

1 whole green onion, finely chopped

1 tsp. dried mint

2 tsp. salt

$^1/_2$ tsp. cayenne

$^1/_2$ tsp. ground black pepper

$^3/_4$ cup fresh lemon juice

1 (16-oz.) jar grape leaves in brine, drained

3 large carrots, cut into diagonal slices

$^3/_4$ cup extra-virgin olive oil

5 cups water

1. In a large bowl, combine long-grain rice, parsley, tomato, yellow onion, green onion, mint, 1 teaspoon salt, cayenne, black pepper, and $^1/_4$ cup lemon juice. Set aside.

2. Cover the bottom of a 2-quart pot with a layer of grape leaves followed by a layer of sliced carrots.

3. Remove stems on remaining leaves and place vein side up on your work surface. Spoon 2 tablespoons filling on each leaf, and roll, tucking in edges as you roll.

4. Stack rolled grape leaves in a circular fashion in the pot. Add remaining $^1/_2$ cup lemon juice, extra-virgin olive oil, and enough water to just cover top of rolled leaves. Season with remaining 1 teaspoon salt, cover, and simmer over medium-low heat for 1 hour, 30 minutes, adding additional water during the cook time as needed.

5. Remove from heat, and let sit for 30 minutes before serving warm or cold.

MEDITERRANEAN MORSEL

Letting the rolled grapes leaves sit for 30 minutes helps ensure the cooked rolls don't fall apart.

Eggplant Casserole (*Moussaka*)

Moussaka is a layered casserole of seasoned eggplant, tomatoes, and sweet sautéed garlic and onions, accompanied by a mild tomato sauce and topped with a toasted breadcrumb crust.

Yield:	Prep time:	Cook time:	Serving size:
1 casserole	40 minutes	1 hour, 20 minutes	$^{1}/_{12}$ casserole
Each serving has:			
228 calories	12g fat	3g saturated fat	8g protein
25g carbohydrate	6g dietary fiber	7mg cholesterol	1,169mg sodium

2 large eggplants

$2^{1}/_{2}$ tsp. salt

$^{1}/_{4}$ cup plus 3 TB. extra-virgin olive oil

2 large white onions, sliced

10 cloves garlic, finely chopped

1 (16-oz.) can chickpeas, rinsed and drained

4 cups plain tomato sauce

1 TB. sugar

1 tsp. ground black pepper

$^{1}/_{2}$ tsp. cayenne

1 tsp. allspice

$^{1}/_{2}$ tsp. nutmeg

1 cup plain breadcrumbs

1 cup shredded Parmesan cheese

1. Slice eggplants into $^{1}/_{4}$-inch slices, sprinkle evenly with 1 teaspoon salt, and place in a strainer to drain for 30 minutes.

2. In a large skillet over medium heat, heat 3 tablespoons extra-virgin olive oil. Add white onions and $^{1}/_{2}$ teaspoon salt, and cook for 5 minutes.

3. Add garlic and chickpeas, and cook for 3 minutes.

4. In a 2-quart pot over medium-low heat, combine tomato sauce, remaining 1 teaspoon salt, sugar, black pepper, cayenne, allspice, and nutmeg. Simmer for 10 minutes.

5. Preheat a large skillet over medium heat, and add remaining $^{1}/_{4}$ cup extra-virgin olive oil.

6. Pat each piece of eggplant dry with a paper towel, and place eggplant in the skillet. Do not overcrowd. Cook for 3 minutes per side, and transfer to a plate lined with paper towels to drain.

7. In a small bowl, combine breadcrumbs and Parmesan cheese. Set aside.

8. Preheat the oven to 400°F.

9. To assemble, ladle a spoonful of tomato sauce on the bottom of a deep casserole dish. Add a layer of eggplant, a layer of tomatoes, a layer of onion mixture, and another layer of sauce. Repeat layering, finishing with a layer of eggplant and tomato sauce. Top with breadcrumb mixture, cover with aluminum foil, and bake for 40 minutes.

10. Remove the foil and let breadcrumbs brown for 5 to 7 minutes.

11. Remove casserole from the oven, and let sit for 20 minutes before serving.

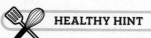 **HEALTHY HINT**

This dish is nutritional because it contains protein from the chickpeas; antioxidants from the garlic, onions, and tomatoes; plus carotenoids from the tomatoes.

Green Beans and Tomatoes

This dish is a great way to prepare protein-filled green beans without any fatty creams. Here, mild onions mingle with sweet tomatoes and a touch of garlic, and all are combined with fresh green beans.

Yield: 8 cups	Prep time: 20 minutes	Cook time: 30 minutes	Serving size: 2 cups
Each serving has:			
206 calories	14g fat	2g saturated fat	4g protein
20g carbohydrate	6g dietary fiber	0mg cholesterol	888mg sodium

$^1/_4$ cup extra-virgin olive oil	$^1/_2$ tsp. ground black pepper
2 medium white onions, chopped	$^1/_2$ tsp. cayenne
$1^1/_2$ tsp. salt	4 cups green beans, trimmed and cut into 1-in. pieces
3 medium tomatoes, chopped	
$^1/_4$ cup minced garlic	

1. In a large, 3-quart pot over medium heat, heat extra-virgin olive oil. Add white onions, and cook for 5 minutes.

2. Add salt, tomatoes, and garlic, and cook for 10 minutes.

3. Add black pepper, cayenne, and green beans, and toss together. Cover and cook for 10 minutes.

4. Serve warm or at room temperature with pita bread.

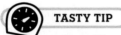 **TASTY TIP**

If you like a little more heat, you could use 1 teaspoon crushed red pepper flakes instead of the cayenne called for in this recipe.

Zucchini Fritters

These zucchini fritters are crunchy on the outside and fluffy on the inside. They're made with fresh zucchini, zesty herbs, and a light batter.

Yield:	Prep time:	Cook time:	Serving size:
12 fritters	15 minutes	10 minutes	1 fritter
Each serving has:			
49 calories	3g fat	1g saturated fat	2g protein
5g carbohydrate	0g dietary fiber	35mg cholesterol	207mg sodium

2 large zucchini, grated

3 whole green onions, finely chopped

$^1/_4$ cup fresh Italian parsley, finely chopped

1 tsp. dried mint

$^1/_2$ tsp. cayenne

1 tsp. salt

$^1/_2$ tsp. ground black pepper

2 large eggs

$^1/_2$ cup all-purpose flour

3 TB. water

1 cup extra-virgin olive oil

1. In a large bowl, combine zucchini, green onions, Italian parsley, mint, cayenne, salt, black pepper, eggs, all-purpose flour, and water.

2. In a 3-quart pot or fryer over high heat, heat extra-virgin olive oil to 325°F.

3. Drop batter into the fryer with a large tablespoon, and fry for 3 minutes per side or until golden brown. Do not overcrowd the pot. Remove fritters from the pot, and place on a plate lined with paper towels. Serve immediately.

Spanakopita

This is a baked casserole-like spinach dish, with a toasted, flaky phyllo crust and cheesy spinach filling.

Yield:	Prep time:	Cook time:	Serving size:
12 slices	30 minutes	35 minutes	1 slice

Each serving has:			
258 calories	19g fat	10g saturated fat	9g protein
13g carbohydrate	1g dietary fiber	80mg cholesterol	556mg sodium

3 TB. extra-virgin olive oil

1 large white onion, chopped

1^1/$_2$ lb. fresh spinach, washed and chopped

^{1}/$_2$ cup fresh parsley, finely chopped

^{1}/$_2$ cup fresh dill, finely chopped

1 lb. ricotta cheese

6 oz. feta cheese, crumbled

^{1}/$_2$ tsp. ground nutmeg

^{1}/$_2$ tsp. ground black pepper

1 tsp. salt

2 large eggs

10 sheets phyllo dough

^{1}/$_2$ cup melted butter

1. In a large skillet over medium heat, heat extra-virgin olive oil. Add white onion, and cook for 5 minutes.

2. Add spinach, and cook for about 5 minutes or until wilted. Remove from heat, and set aside to cool.

3. In a large bowl, combine cooked onions and spinach, parsley, dill, ricotta cheese, feta cheese, nutmeg, black pepper, salt, and eggs.

4. Preheat the oven to 400°F.

5. Cut phyllo sheets to fit in a 9×13-inch pan.

6. Layer 10 sheets of phyllo dough, brushing each layer with melted butter, on the bottom of the pan. Spread spinach filling evenly over phyllo sheets. Layer another 10 sheets of phyllo dough on top of filling, brushing each layer with melted butter as you stack them.

7. Using a sharp knife, score top 2 or 3 layers of phyllo dough into 12 even pieces. Bake for 25 minutes or until golden brown.

8. Remove from the oven, and let stand for 20 minutes before serving.

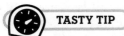 **TASTY TIP**

> If your only option is to use frozen spinach in the **Spanakopita,** be sure to squeeze out as much of the water as possible. Otherwise, you'll get a soggy finished dish.

Zesty Flatbread Pizza

I love making this recipe when I'm in the mood for pizza but not for all that melted cheese. The peppery arugula and the pungent goat cheese flavor this pizza in a very unique way.

Yield:	Prep time:	Cook time:	Serving size:
1 (12-inch) pizza	15 minutes	10 minutes	1/8 pizza

Each serving has:			
214 calories	15g fat	5g saturated fat	6g protein
15g carbohydrate	1g dietary fiber	14mg cholesterol	439mg sodium

1 (12-in.) premade flatbread	5 oz. goat cheese
3 TB. extra-virgin olive oil	12 kalamata olives, sliced
1/2 tsp. salt	2 cups fresh arugula
1/2 tsp. ground black pepper	3 TB. balsamic vinegar
2 roma tomatoes, thinly sliced	

1. Preheat the oven to 400°F.

2. Place flatbread on a pizza pan or baking sheet. Drizzle with 2 tablespoons extra-virgin olive oil, and sprinkle with salt and black pepper.

3. Evenly distribute roma tomato slices over flatbread, crumble goat cheese on top, and sprinkle with kalamata olives. Bake for 10 minutes.

4. Meanwhile, in a small bowl, toss arugula, remaining 1 tablespoon extra-virgin olive oil, and balsamic vinegar.

5. Remove pizza from the oven, and cut into 8 slices. Top with arugula, and serve warm.

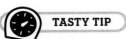 **TASTY TIP**

> If you don't like goat cheese, you can replace it with feta cheese.

Mediterranean Grilled Cheese Sandwiches

This recipe makes a quick and easy grilled cheese sandwich, but one with a whole lot of flavor, thanks to the three different cheeses used plus the tangy sun-dried tomatoes.

Yield:	Prep time:	Cook time:	Serving size:
4 sandwiches	10 minutes	8 minutes	1 sandwich

Each serving has:			
657 calories	48g fat	23g saturated fat	30g protein
26g carbohydrate	2g dietary fiber	110mg cholesterol	1,061mg sodium

8 pieces rustic loaf bread

8 oz. Brie cheese, cut into 8 slices

4 slices Havarti cheese

$^1/_2$ cup fresh basil, finely chopped

$^1/_2$ cup sun-dried tomatoes, finely chopped

1 tsp. ground black pepper

4 slices Colby jack cheese

4 TB. extra-virgin olive oil

1. Place 4 slices bread on your work surface, top each slice with 2 slices of Brie cheese and 1 slice Havarti cheese.

2. Evenly divide basil and sun-dried tomato among sandwiches, sprinkle with ground black pepper, and top with 1 slice of Colby jack cheese each. Cover each sandwich with remaining slices of bread.

3. Preheat a large skillet or griddle over medium heat. Add 2 tablespoons extra-virgin olive oil, and cook sandwiches for 4 minutes on one side.

4. Drizzle remaining 2 tablespoons extra-virgin olive oil over sandwiches, flip them over, and cook for 4 more minutes.

5. Remove from heat, and serve warm.

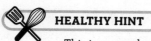 **HEALTHY HINT**

This is a very decadent sandwich. If you're trying to save some calories, opt for a half sandwich with a side of mixed greens dressed with balsamic vinegar, salt, and black pepper.

Fried Eggplant and Cauliflower Sandwiches

These sandwiches were one of my mother's go-to dishes when she didn't want to do a lot of cooking. They're fast and easy—and they taste great.

Yield:	Prep time:	Cook time:	Serving size:
3 sandwiches	40 minutes	20 minutes	$^1/_2$ sandwich

Each serving has:			
435 calories	25g fat	18g saturated fat	9g protein
46g carbohydrate	9g dietary fiber	1mg cholesterol	744mg sodium

1 large eggplant	2 tsp. seven spices
$1^1/_2$ tsp. salt	3 pitas
1 medium head cauliflower	6 TB. Yogurt Spread (*Labne;* recipe
2 large potatoes, peeled	in Chapter 3)
6 cups vegetable oil	

1. Slice eggplant into $^1/_4$-inch slices, sprinkle evenly with $^1/_2$ teaspoon salt, and place in a strainer to drain for 30 minutes.

2. Cut cauliflower into florets, and cut potatoes into french fries.

3. In a large 3-quart pot over high heat, heat vegetable oil to 365°F.

4. Pat dry eggplant slices, carefully place in the pot, and fry for 3 minutes per side. Remove from the pot, and place on a plate lined with paper towels to drain. Season with 1 teaspoon seven spices.

5. Carefully place cauliflower in the pot, and fry for 6 minutes. Remove from the pot, and place on a plate lined with paper towels to drain. Season with remaining 1 teaspoon seven spices and $^1/_2$ teaspoon salt.

6. Carefully place potato strips in the pot, and fry for 8 minutes. Remove from the pot, and place on a plate lined with paper towels to drain. Season with remaining $^1/_2$ teaspoon salt.

7. Lay out 1 piece of pita; spread with 2 tablespoons Yogurt Spread (*Labne*); and add a few pieces of eggplant, cauliflower, and potatoes down middle of pita. Roll pita into a sandwich, cut in half, and serve.

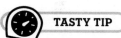 **TASTY TIP**

If you like the taste of mint, try adding some freshly chopped mint to the sandwich before serving.

Great Grain, Rice, and Bean Dishes

In This Chapter

- Hearty bulgur dishes
- Pleasing pilafs
- Beneficial bean dishes

Any recipe can seem complicated if you don't have the ingredients on hand or the time to fully prepare the dish. That's why, in the earlier chapters in this book, I emphasize the need to plan ahead. Having a well-stocked pantry can broaden your options when it comes to mealtime. Even cooking ahead is a great idea.

You can make all the recipes in this chapter ahead of time. For example, you can make one or two dishes on Sunday and store them in individual serving containers in the refrigerator. Then, when you're ready, you can just grab and go. Planning and cooking ahead keeps you from going to fast-food places at lunch or dinner and eating something that won't benefit you in any way.

Many of the recipes in this chapter focus on grains and beans. Beans are one of the healthiest foods you can eat, full of nutrients, minerals, fiber, and protein—it's almost everything you need in a tiny little package. Not only are beans nutritional, but they also fill you up without the need for meat because of their complex carbohydrates. Whole grains are almost as good for you, so it just makes sense to make these two foods a key part of your diet.

Bulgur with Seasoned Lamb

This lamb dish, with seasoned bulgur and sweet onions, brings back memories from my grandmother's house.

Yield:	Prep time:	Cook time:	Serving size:
8 cups	20 minutes	40 minutes	1 cup

Each serving has:			
423 calories	25g fat	10g saturated fat	30g protein
20g carbohydrate	4g dietary fiber	93mg cholesterol	782mg sodium

2 ($1^1/_2$-lb.) lamb shanks

8 cups water

2 large yellow onions, chopped

2 bay leaves

1 (3-in.) cinnamon stick

3 whole cloves

2 tsp. salt

3 TB. extra-virgin olive oil

1 (16-oz.) can chickpeas, rinsed and drained

$^1/_2$ tsp. cinnamon

$^1/_2$ tsp. allspice

1 tsp. ground black pepper

2 cups bulgur wheat, grind #2

1. In a pressure cooker over medium heat, add lamb shanks, water, half of yellow onions, bay leaves, cinnamon stick, cloves, and 1 teaspoon salt. Bring to a simmer, skimming off any surface foam, and cook for about 10 minutes.

2. Reduce heat to low, cover, and cook for 30 minutes.

3. Release pressure from the pressure cooker, and let cool for about 30 minutes before removing the lid.

4. Transfer lamb shanks to a plate, and set aside until cool enough to handle. Remove bones from shanks, and cut meat into bite-size pieces.

5. Remove and discard bay leaves and cinnamon stick from lamb broth in the pressure cooker.

6. In a large 3-quart pot over medium heat, heat extra-virgin olive oil. Add remaining half of yellow onions, and cook for 5 minutes.

7. Add chickpeas, lamb chunks, cinnamon, allspice, black pepper, remaining 1 teaspoon salt, and 4 cups lamb broth from the pressure cooker, and simmer for 5 minutes.

8. Add bulgur wheat, and cook for 2 minutes. Remove from heat, cover, and let sit for 5 minutes. Uncover, fluff bulgur with a fork, cover, and let sit for 5 more minutes. Serve warm.

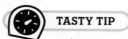 **TASTY TIP**

If you're not a fan of lamb, you can replace it with chicken drumsticks instead.

Bulgur Chickpea Pilaf

In this vegetarian pilaf, full of fiber and protein, earthy bulgur wheat combines with toasted vermicelli noodles.

Yield:	Prep time:	Cook time:	Serving size:
8 cups	10 minutes	15 minutes	1 cup

Each serving has:			
207 calories	6g fat	1g saturated fat	6g protein
33g carbohydrate	5g dietary fiber	0mg cholesterol	911mg sodium

3 TB. extra-virgin olive oil

1 large yellow onion, finely chopped

1 cup vermicelli noodles

1 (16-oz.) can chickpeas, rinsed and drained

4 cups vegetable broth

1 tsp. cinnamon

1$^{1}/_{2}$ tsp. salt

$^{1}/_{2}$ tsp. ground black pepper

2 cups bulgur wheat, grind #2

1. Preheat a large, 3-quart pot over medium heat. Add extra-virgin olive oil and yellow onion, and cook for 5 minutes.

2. Add vermicelli noodles, and cook for 3 minutes.

3. Add chickpeas, vegetable broth, cinnamon, salt, and black pepper, and cook for 5 minutes.

4. Add bulgur wheat, and cook for 2 minutes. Remove from heat, cover, and let sit for 5 minutes. Uncover, fluff bulgur with a fork, cover, and let sit for 5 more minutes. Serve warm with Greek yogurt.

Bulgur Tomato Pilaf

In this dish, earthy bulgur is simmered in a meaty tomato sauce filled with chunks of tomatoes and onions.

Yield:	Prep time:	Cook time:	Serving size:
6 cups	20 minutes	27 minutes	1 cup

Each serving has:			
285 calories	16g fat	4g saturated fat	17g protein
20g carbohydrate	5g dietary fiber	44mg cholesterol	1,061mg sodium

1 lb. ground beef	1 tsp. ground black pepper
3 TB. extra-virgin olive oil	2 cups plain tomato sauce
1 large yellow onion, finely chopped	2 cups water
2 medium tomatoes, diced	2 cups bulgur wheat, grind #2
1¹/₂ tsp. salt	

1. In a large, 3-quart pot over medium heat, brown beef for 5 minutes, breaking up chunks with a wooden spoon.

2. Add extra-virgin olive oil and yellow onion, and cook for 5 minutes.

3. Stir in tomatoes, salt, and black pepper, and cook for 5 minutes.

4. Add tomato sauce and water, and simmer for 10 minutes.

5. Add bulgur wheat, and cook for 2 minutes. Remove from heat, cover, and let sit for 5 minutes. Uncover, fluff bulgur with a fork, cover, and let sit for 5 more minutes.

6. Serve warm.

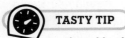 **TASTY TIP**

If you like things spicy, add some crushed red pepper flakes to this recipe. Or serve with a finely chopped jalapeño pepper on top.

Freekeh Pilaf

Smoky green wheat freekeh has a very earthy, robust flavor that's delicious when combined with fresh herbs, as in this dish.

Yield:	Prep time:	Cook time:	Serving size:
6 cups	20 minutes	1 hour, 5 minutes	1 cup

Each serving has:			
395 calories	11g fat	1g saturated fat	16g protein
61g carbohydrate	14g dietary fiber	0mg cholesterol	1,365mg sodium

3 TB. extra-virgin olive oil	1 tsp. paprika
1 large white onion, chopped	2 cups freekeh wheat
2 cups crimini mushrooms, rinsed and sliced	6 cups vegetable or chicken broth
2 TB. minced garlic	3 cups fresh baby spinach, coarsely chopped
1½ tsp. salt	2 TB. fresh thyme
1 TB. ground coriander	2 TB. fresh Italian parsley, chopped
1 tsp. ground black pepper	

1. In a large, 3-quart pot over medium heat, heat extra-virgin olive oil. Add white onion, and cook for 5 minutes.

2. Add crimini mushrooms, garlic, and salt, and cook for 5 minutes.

3. Add coriander, black pepper, paprika, and freekeh, and cook for 2 minutes.

4. Stir in vegetable broth, cover, reduce heat to low, and simmer for 40 minutes.

5. Uncover, and stir in spinach, thyme, and Italian parsley. Cover and cook for 15 minutes. Remove from heat, fluff with a fork, cover, and let stand for 15 minutes. Serve warm.

Spiced Tomato No-Bake Pilaf

I love this pilaf during the summertime because it's the perfect dish in which to use sweet, vine-ripened tomatoes. The nutty bulgur paired with the sweet tomatoes and abundance of herbs and spices—this pilaf leaves your taste buds completely satisfied.

Yield:	Prep time:	Serving size:	
6 cups	15 minutes	1 cup	
Each serving has:			
192 calories	13g fat	2g saturated fat	4g protein
19g carbohydrate	6g dietary fiber	0mg cholesterol	604mg sodium

1 medium white onion, chopped	$^1/_2$ tsp. cayenne
$^1/_2$ cup fresh basil	2 TB. paprika
$^1/_2$ cup fresh mint	$1^1/_2$ tsp. salt
$^1/_2$ tsp. ground allspice	$^1/_2$ tsp. ground black pepper
$^1/_2$ tsp. ground cumin	1 cup bulgur wheat, grind #1
$^1/_2$ tsp. ground coriander	6 large ripe red tomatoes, finely diced
$^1/_4$ tsp. ground nutmeg	1 cup fresh Italian parsley, finely chopped
$^1/_4$ tsp. ground cloves	
$^1/_4$ tsp. ground cinnamon	4 whole green onions, finely chopped
$^1/_2$ tsp. ground sage	$^1/_3$ cup extra-virgin olive oil
1 tsp. dried thyme	

1. In a food processor fitted with a chopping blade, blend white onion, basil, and mint for 30 seconds.

2. Add allspice, cumin, coriander, nutmeg, cloves, cinnamon, sage, thyme, cayenne, paprika, salt, black pepper, and bulgur wheat, and blend for 1 minute.

3. Transfer bulgur mixture to a bowl. Add tomatoes, Italian parsley, green onions, and extra-virgin olive oil, and toss. Let sit for 15 to 20 minutes.

4. Serve cold or at room temperature with pita bread.

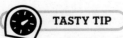 **TASTY TIP**

The longer you let this dish sit, the better it tastes as the bulgur absorbs all the flavors. If you find it to be a little dry the next day, you can add some fresh chopped tomatoes and a few tablespoons of extra-virgin olive oil.

Pumpkin Kibbeh

This kibbeh has a very distinct flavor, thanks to the sweet pumpkin and fragrant spices.

Yield:	Prep time:	Cook time:	Serving size:
12 kibbeh	40 minutes	1 hour, 20 minutes	1 kibbeh

Each serving has:			
199 calories	11g fat	1g saturated fat	5g protein
22g carbohydrate	4g dietary fiber	0mg cholesterol	450mg sodium

1 medium sugar pumpkin

2 cups bulgur wheat, grind #1

2 cups water

1 large yellow onion, coarsely chopped

2 tsp. salt

$^1/_2$ tsp. ground black pepper

$^1/_2$ tsp. ground cinnamon

$^1/_2$ tsp. ground allspice

$^1/_2$ tsp. ground ginger

$^1/_2$ tsp. paprika

$^1/_2$ tsp. turmeric

1 cup all-purpose flour

3 TB. extra-virgin olive oil

$^1/_2$ cup walnuts, chopped

$^1/_2$ cup pine nuts

1 tsp. seven spices

1 (16-oz.) can chickpeas, rinsed and drained

Olive oil spray

1. Preheat the oven to 450°F.

2. Cut sugar pumpkin in half, place cut side down on a baking sheet, and bake for 45 minutes.

3. In a large bowl, combine bulgur wheat and water, and set aside for 20 minutes.

4. When pumpkin is done baking, remove seeds and stringy pulp, and scoop out pumpkin meat (about 4 cups).

5. In a food processor fitted with a chopping blade, blend $^1/_2$ of yellow onion for 30 seconds.

6. Add pumpkin, and blend for 30 seconds.

7. Add bulgur, salt, black pepper, cinnamon, allspice, ginger, paprika, and turmeric, and blend for 1 minute. (You can do this in batches if your food processor won't hold all of bulgur and pumpkin at once.)

8. Transfer mixture to a large bowl, and knead all-purpose flour into pumpkin-bulgur mix for about 3 minutes.

9. In a medium skillet over medium heat, heat extra-virgin olive oil. Add remaining yellow onion, and cook for 5 minutes.

10. Add walnuts, pine nuts, and seven spices, and cook for 3 minutes.

11. Add chickpeas, and cook for 2 minutes.

12. Form pumpkin dough into 24 (3-inch) patties. Spoon 2 tablespoons chickpea mixture on 12 patties, and use remaining 12 patties to cover. Seal patties around chickpea mixture.

13. Spray sealed kibbeh with olive oil spray, and spray a baking sheet, too. Place kibbeh on the baking sheet, and bake for 25 minutes. Remove, let cool slightly, and serve warm.

 MEDITERRANEAN MORSEL

Kibbeh is a dough made using bulgur wheat and either meat or a puréed vegetable. It's eaten raw, baked, or fried and usually has a filling.

Zucchini and Brown Rice

Zucchini is a very versatile vegetable. In this dish, it takes on a new character when paired with the earthy brown rice, zesty dill, and tangy artichoke hearts.

Yield:	Prep time:	Cook time:	Serving size:
8 cups	20 minutes	50 minutes	1 cup
Each serving has:			
121 calories	5g fat	1g saturated fat	4g protein
15g carbohydrate	2g dietary fiber	0mg cholesterol	673mg sodium

2 TB. extra-virgin olive oil

2 large zucchini, diced

1 (16-oz.) can artichoke hearts, rinsed and drained

1 TB. fresh dill

1 tsp. ground black pepper

1 tsp. salt

4 cups chicken or vegetable broth

2 cups basmati brown rice

1. In a large, 3-quart pot over medium heat, heat extra-virgin olive oil. Add zucchini, and cook for 3 minutes.

2. Add artichoke hearts, and cook for 2 minutes.

3. Add dill, black pepper, salt, and chicken broth, and bring to a simmer. Stir in basmati brown rice, cover, reduce heat to low, and cook for 40 minutes.

4. Remove from heat, uncover, fluff with a fork, cover, and let sit for another 15 minutes. Serve with Greek yogurt.

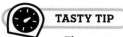

TASTY TIP

The secret to getting a fluffy rice or pilaf is the last step: you must let it sit for 15 minutes after cooking. This helps the grain steam and not stick together.

Lentils and Rice (*Mujaddara* with Rice)

This filling dish is full of fiber and protein. The earthy lentils and rice provide all the fiber and protein with a nice amount of seasoning to liven up the dish.

Yield:	Prep time:	Cook time:	Serving size:
6 cups	20 minutes	1 hour, 10 minutes	1 cup
Each serving has:			
204 calories	10g fat	1g saturated fat	7g protein
23g carbohydrate	6g dietary fiber	0mg cholesterol	780mg sodium

¼ cup extra-virgin olive oil	6 cups water
1 large yellow onion, finely chopped	1 cup long-grain rice or brown rice
2 tsp. salt	1 TB. cumin
2 cups green or brown lentils, picked over and rinsed	

1. In a large, 3-quart pot over medium-low heat, heat extra-virgin olive oil. Add yellow onion and 1 teaspoon salt, and cook, stirring intermittently, for 10 minutes.

2. Add green lentils and water, and cook, stirring intermittently, for 20 minutes.

3. Stir in long-grain rice, remaining 1 teaspoon salt, and cumin. Cover and cook, stirring intermittently, for 40 minutes.

4. Serve warm or at room temperature with tzatziki sauce or a Mediterranean salad.

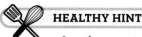

HEALTHY HINT

Lentils are a nice source of protein, fiber, and iron, and brown rice is a good source of complex carbohydrates. This dish is a great example of what you should be eating every day—all in one plate!

Lentils and Bulgur Wheat Pilaf
(*Mujaddara Hamra*)

This lentil pilaf contains onions, onions, and more onions. But the flavor isn't like you imagine—it's actually sweet because the onions are slowly cooked to caramelize them. The lentils and bulgur soak up all the flavor and add a hint of earthiness.

Yield:	Prep time:	Cook time:	Serving size:
6 cups	20 minutes	1 hour	1 cup

Each serving has:			
331 calories	19g fat	3g saturated fat	9g protein
35g carbohydrate	9g dietary fiber	0mg cholesterol	785mg sodium

$\frac{1}{2}$ cup extra-virgin olive oil

2 large yellow onions, chopped

2 tsp. salt

2 cups green or brown lentils, picked over and rinsed

6 cups water

1 TB. cumin

1 tsp. ground black pepper

1 cup bulgur wheat, grind #2

3 cups pearl onions, peeled

1. In a large, 3-quart pot over medium-low heat, heat $\frac{1}{4}$ cup extra-virgin olive oil. Add yellow onions and 1 teaspoon salt, and cook, stirring intermittently, for 20 minutes or until onions are dark brown but not burned.

2. Add green lentils, water, remaining 1 teaspoon salt, and cumin, and cook, stirring intermittently, for 40 minutes.

3. Stir in black pepper and bulgur wheat, cover, and cook for 5 minutes. Remove from heat, uncover, fluff with a fork, cover, and set aside for 10 minutes.

4. In a large skillet over medium-low heat, heat remaining $\frac{1}{4}$ cup extra-virgin olive oil. Add pearl onions, and cook, stirring intermittently, for 15 minutes.

5. To serve, spoon a few spoonfuls of lentil pilaf onto a plate and top with pearl onions.

Snacks, Sauces, and More

There's nothing like a satisfying snack that hits the spot just when you need something to carry you over to the next meal. In addition, it's important that the snack is healthy and doesn't derail your new healthy diet and lifestyle.

In Part 4, I give you a selection of Mediterranean-inspired dips, appetizers, breads, and sauces so you can prepare healthy snacks *before* you get hungry and resort to something not so good for you.

Delightful Dips and Spreads

When you think of Mediterranean food, perhaps one of the first foods that comes to mind is hummus. Hummus is a real power food, filled with protein, complex carbohydrates, antioxidants, and flavor. It's also very versatile. You can eat it as a side dish, as a dip with veggies, as a spread for your sandwich, as a snack with crackers, or as a main dish topped with meat or cooked vegetables. It's also a great recipe for flavor variations, and you'll find several versions in this chapter. But don't be afraid to experiment and make your own hummus varieties. Try adding your favorite herb, or instead of using fresh garlic, try using roasted garlic.

In addition, this chapter's other recipes are also full of robust flavor. What's more, not only are they flavorful, they're also full of nutritious ingredients that are good for you, not just empty calories. Dress up a turkey sandwich using the Roasted Red Pepper and Sun-Dried Tomato Tapenade instead of mayonnaise, for example, and your taste buds will be delighted.

In This Chapter

- Hearty hummus
- Delectable dips
- Sensational spreads

Traditional Hummus

I love the smooth texture of this hummus recipe. The nutty flavor from the sesame seed paste combined with the tangy lemon flavor and a hint of garlic gives this hummus an almost three-dimensional flavor.

Yield:	Prep time:	Serving size:	
2 cups	10 minutes	2 tablespoons	
Each serving has:			
78 calories	6g fat	1g saturated fat	2g protein
5g carbohydrate	1g dietary fiber	0mg cholesterol	124mg sodium

1 (15-oz.) can chickpeas, rinsed and drained

3 cloves garlic, peeled

$^1/_4$ cup fresh lemon juice

$^1/_2$ tsp. salt

$^1/_4$ cup plain Greek yogurt

$^1/_2$ cup tahini paste

2 TB. extra-virgin olive oil

3 fresh mint leaves

1. In a food processor fitted with a chopping blade, blend chickpeas, garlic, lemon juice, and salt for 2 minutes or until smooth. Scrape down the sides of the food processor bowl with a rubber spatula.

2. Add Greek yogurt, tahini paste, and extra-virgin olive oil and blend for 1 minute or until creamy and well combined.

3. Add mint leaves, and pulse for 30 seconds or until you see little specks of green mint throughout.

4. Serve, or refrigerate for up to 1 week.

 MEDITERRANEAN MORSEL

Presentation is a big part of eating in the Mediterranean culture, and serving your food in appealing dishes with pretty garnish is a must. To serve hummus, spread it onto a nice plate, garnish with fresh sprigs of parsley or mint, sprinkle with paprika, and drizzle with extra-virgin olive oil. The olive oil not only makes the hummus look nice, it also adds flavor, keeps the hummus moist, and prevents it from drying out.

Hummus with Meat

This protein-filled hummus is amazingly easy to make. The combination of the spiced ground beef with the smooth and tangy flavor of the hummus pair well together.

Yield:	Prep time:	Cook time:	Serving size:
4 cups	20 minutes	15 minutes	$^1/_2$ cup

Each serving has:			
281 calories	22g fat	3g saturated fat	11g protein
12g carbohydrate	3g dietary fiber	17mg cholesterol	412mg sodium

$^1/_2$ lb. lean ground beef

$^1/_2$ tsp. salt

$^1/_2$ tsp. ground black pepper

$^1/_2$ tsp. seven spices

1 TB. extra-virgin olive oil

$^1/_2$ cup pine nuts

1 batch Traditional Hummus (recipe earlier in this chapter)

$^1/_2$ tsp. paprika

2 TB. fresh parsley, chopped

1. In a small saucepan over medium heat, brown ground beef and salt for about 5 minutes, breaking up chunks with a wooden spoon.

2. Stir in black pepper and seven spices, and cook for 1 minute. Remove from heat.

3. In another small saucepan over low heat, heat extra-virgin olive oil. Add pine nuts, and cook, stirring, for about 2 minutes or until golden brown. Remove from heat.

4. Spread Traditional Hummus to $^1/_2$ inch thickness on a serving plate, and sprinkle with paprika. Evenly spoon meat over center of hummus, evenly top beef with toasted pine nuts, and sprinkle with parsley.

5. Serve warm or at room temperature with pita bread or pita chips.

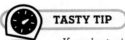 **TASTY TIP**

If you're trying to incorporate more fiber and protein into your diet, this is the perfect recipe to do just that. The addition of meat and pine nuts in the hummus boosts the amount of both.

Cilantro Jalapeño Hummus

I call this my southwestern hummus—it's my alternative to salsa. The cilantro and jalapeño really bring out the southwest flavor and add a little kick to the nutty tahini flavor.

Yield:	Prep time:	Serving size:	
2 cups	10 minutes	2 tablespoons	
Each serving has:			
73 calories	6g fat	1g saturated fat	2g protein
4g carbohydrate	1g dietary fiber	0mg cholesterol	119mg sodium

1 (15-oz.) can chickpeas, rinsed and drained	$^1/_2$ cup tahini paste
3 cloves garlic, peeled	2 TB. extra-virgin olive oil
$^1/_4$ cup fresh lime juice	$^1/_2$ jalapeño, ribs and seeds removed
$^1/_2$ tsp. salt	$^1/_3$ cup cilantro leaves, finely chopped
$^1/_4$ cup plain Greek yogurt	

1. In a food processor fitted with a chopping blade, blend chickpeas, garlic, lime juice, and salt for 2 minutes or until smooth. Scrape down the sides of the food processor bowl with a rubber spatula.

2. Add Greek yogurt, tahini paste, and extra-virgin olive oil, and blend for 1 minute or until creamy and well combined.

3. Add jalapeño, and pulse for 30 seconds.

4. Add cilantro, and pulse 10 times.

5. Serve with tortilla chips.

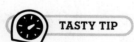 **TASTY TIP**

For a spicy kick, include the jalapeño seeds when blending. They contain most of the heat that's in a jalapeño pepper.

Roasted Red Pepper Hummus

This hummus variation has a smoky flavor with a hint of sweetness from the roasted red pepper. Adding a little cayenne gives it a bit of kick at the end of each bite.

Yield:	Prep time:	Cook time:	Serving size:
2 cups	15 minutes	20 minutes	2 tablespoons

Each serving has:			
85 calories	7g fat	1g saturated fat	2g protein
5g carbohydrate	2g dietary fiber	0mg cholesterol	119mg sodium

1 large red bell pepper	2 TB. plain Greek yogurt
1 (15-oz.) can chickpeas, rinsed and drained	$^1/_2$ cup plus 2 TB. tahini paste
3 cloves garlic, peeled	2 TB. extra-virgin olive oil
$^1/_4$ cup fresh lemon juice	1 tsp. paprika
$^1/_2$ tsp. salt	$^1/_2$ tsp. cayenne

1. Preheat a grill top or a grill to medium heat.

2. Place red bell pepper on the grill, and cook on all sides for about 20 minutes or until charred. Immediately place pepper on a plate, cover with plastic wrap, let cool for 10 minutes.

3. When pepper is cool enough to handle, peel off skin. (It's okay if it doesn't all come off.) Remove stalk and seeds.

4. In a food processor fitted with a chopping blade, blend roasted red pepper, chickpeas, garlic, lemon juice, and salt for 2 minutes or until smooth. Scrape down the sides of the food processor bowl with a rubber spatula.

5. Add Greek yogurt, tahini paste, extra-virgin olive oil, paprika, and cayenne, blend for 1 minute or until creamy and well combined.

6. Serve with pita chips, or refrigerate for up to 1 week.

 MEDITERRANEAN MORSEL

If you don't have time to grill a red bell pepper, you can use roasted red bell peppers from a jar. Or the next time you have the grill going, roast a few extra bell peppers, peel, remove the seeds, and freeze them in individual bags for use later.

White Bean Hummus

This has the smooth flavor of hummus but with a variation from the usual chickpeas. The cannellini beans give it a mild flavor with the underlying pungency of the Parmesan cheese.

Yield:	Prep time:	Serving size:	
2 cups	10 minutes	2 tablespoons	
Each serving has:			
111 calories	9g fat	2g saturated fat	3g protein
5g carbohydrate	1g dietary fiber	3mg cholesterol	238mg sodium

1 (15-oz.) can cannellini beans, rinsed and drained

1 TB. minced garlic

3 TB. lemon juice

1 tsp. salt

$1/3$ cup tahini paste

$1/2$ cup grated Parmesan cheese

6 TB. extra-virgin olive oil

2 TB. fresh basil, chopped

$1/2$ tsp. fresh ground black pepper

3 TB. chopped sun-dried tomatoes

6 kalamata olives

1. In a food processor fitted with a chopping blade, blend cannellini beans, garlic, lemon juice, and salt for 2 minutes or until smooth.

2. Add tahini paste, Parmesan cheese, and 3 tablespoons extra-virgin olive oil, and blend for 1 minute.

3. Add basil and black pepper, and pulse 10 times.

4. Spread hummus on a plate, and drizzle with remaining 3 tablespoons extra-virgin olive oil. Garnish hummus with sun-dried tomatoes and kalamata olives.

5. Serve with pita bread or crackers.

Volcano Feta

This feta dip is tangy, thanks to the feta, and has a huge kick, thanks to the crushed red pepper flakes. A hint of smoky flavor, thanks to the roasted red pepper, rounds out this dip you can serve on a cracker or in a sandwich.

Yield:	Prep time:	Cook time:	Serving size:
2 cups	15 minutes	20 minutes	2 tablespoons

Each serving has:			
75 calories	6g fat	3g saturated fat	3g protein
3g carbohydrate	1g dietary fiber	13mg cholesterol	230mg sodium

1 large red bell pepper	2 TB. crushed red pepper flakes
1 cup feta cheese, crumbled	$^1/_2$ tsp. ground black pepper
1 cup sun-dried tomatoes, chopped	3 TB. extra-virgin olive oil

1. Preheat a grill top or a grill to medium heat.

2. Place red bell pepper on the grill, and cook on all sides for about 20 minutes or until charred. Immediately place pepper on a plate, cover with plastic wrap, let cool for 10 minutes.

3. When pepper is cool enough to handle, peel off skin. (It's okay if it doesn't all come off.) Remove stalk and seeds, and finely dice.

4. In a medium bowl, combine roasted red pepper, feta cheese, sun-dried tomatoes, crushed red pepper flakes, black pepper, and extra-virgin olive oil.

5. Serve immediately, or refrigerate for up to 1 week.

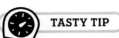 **TASTY TIP**

This feta dip is fantastic as a spread on sandwiches with chicken or grilled vegetables. It adds an extra punch of flavor you'll love.

Muhammara **Spread**

This spicy hot pepper spread has nutty undertones from the toasted walnuts. Each bite boasts an array of flavors due to the paprika, molasses, cumin, and garlic.

Yield:	Prep time:	Cook time:	Serving size:
2 cups	20 minutes	30 minutes	2 tablespoons

Each serving has:			
114 calories	9g fat	1g saturated fat	2g protein
7g carbohydrate	2g dietary fiber	0mg cholesterol	159mg sodium

2 large red bell peppers	3 TB. pomegranate molasses
1 1/2 cups walnuts	1 TB. paprika
1/4 cup plain breadcrumbs	1 tsp. cumin
1 TB. crushed red pepper flakes	1 tsp. salt
3 cloves garlic	1/2 tsp. ground black pepper
3 TB. lemon juice	2 TB. extra-virgin olive oil

1. Preheat a grill top or a grill to medium heat.

2. Place red bell peppers on the grill, and cook on all sides for about 20 minutes or until charred. Immediately place peppers on a plate, cover with plastic wrap, let cool for 10 minutes.

3. Preheat the oven to 450°F.

4. When peppers are cool enough to handle, peel off skin. (It's okay if it doesn't all come off.) Remove stalks and seeds.

5. Spread walnuts evenly on a baking sheet, and bake for 7 minutes or until they're lightly toasted. Be sure not to burn them.

6. In a food processor fitted with a chopping blade, blend roasted red bell peppers, toasted walnuts, breadcrumbs, crushed red pepper flakes, garlic, lemon juice, pomegranate molasses, paprika, cumin, salt, black pepper, and extra-virgin olive oil for 2 minutes or until well combined, intermittently scraping down the sides of the food processor bowl with a rubber spatula.

7. Serve cold or at room temperature.

MEDITERRANEAN MORSEL

Pomegranate molasses is made of pomegranate seeds that have been cooked down. It's tangy and pungent. You usually can find it in the ethnic cuisine aisle of your local grocery store or at your local Turkish, Greek, or Middle Eastern market.

Eggplant Dip (*Mutabal*)

This recipe is sometimes called baba ganoush, but the correct name is mutabal. Regardless of what you call it, it's an amazingly tasty dish. Roasted eggplant, with its smoky flavor, is combined with toasty tahini paste and a slight tang from the lemon juice.

Yield:	Prep time:	Cook time:	Serving size:
3 cups	20 minutes	40 minutes	2 tablespoons

Each serving has:			
26 calories	2g fat	0g saturated fat	1g protein
1g carbohydrate	1g dietary fiber	0mg cholesterol	38mg sodium

2 large eggplants	$^3/_4$ tsp. salt
$^1/_2$ cup tahini paste	1 tsp. paprika
3 TB. lemon juice	$^1/_3$ cup pomegranate seeds (optional)
2 TB. plain Greek yogurt	3 TB. extra-virgin olive oil
1 TB. minced garlic	

1. Preheat a grill top or a grill to medium-low heat.

2. Place eggplants on the grill, and roast on all sides for 40 minutes, turning every 5 minutes. Immediately place eggplants on a plate, cover with plastic wrap, let cool for 15 minutes.

3. Remove eggplant stems, and peel off as much skin as possible. (It's okay if it doesn't all come off.)

4. In a food processor fitted with a chopping blade, pulse eggplant 7 times. Transfer eggplant to a medium bowl.

5. Add tahini paste, lemon juice, Greek yogurt, garlic, and salt to eggplant, and stir for about 1 minute. Taste and adjust salt if needed.

6. To serve, spread mutabal on a flat serving plate, sprinkle with paprika, decorate the plate with pomegranate seeds (if using), and drizzle with extra-virgin olive oil. Serve at room temperature.

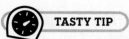 **TASTY TIP**

If you find that the texture of your Eggplant Dip is too runny, try adding an extra 1 or 2 tablespoons tahini paste. It serves as a thickener.

Olive Tapenade

This tapenade is so versatile. I like eating it with crackers or spooning it over baked fish. Either way, it adds a pungent brine flavor with the freshness of herbs.

Yield:	Prep time:	Serving size:	
2 cups	5 minutes	2 tablespoons	
Each serving has:			
79 calories	7g fat	1g saturated fat	0g protein
3g carbohydrate	1g dietary fiber	0mg cholesterol	464mg sodium

1 cup black kalamata olives, pitted	2 TB. capers, drained
1 cup green manzanilla olives, pitted	1 TB. fresh lemon juice
1 tsp. minced garlic	2 TB. extra-virgin olive oil
1 TB. fresh rosemary, finely chopped	

1. In a food processor fitted with a chopping blade, pulse kalamata olives, manzanilla olives, and garlic 10 times. Scrape down the sides of the food processor bowl with a rubber spatula.

2. Add rosemary, capers, lemon juice, and extra-virgin olive oil, and pulse 5 times.

3. Serve immediately, or refrigerate for up to 1 week.

Roasted Red Pepper and Sun-Dried Tomato Tapenade

This zesty tapenade combines the smoky flavor of roasted red peppers, the sweet flavor of sun-dried tomatoes, and the fresh flavor of green herbs.

Yield:	Prep time:	Cook time:	Serving size:
2 cups	15 minutes	20 minutes	2 tablespoons

Each serving has:			
26 calories	2g fat	0g saturated fat	1g protein
2g carbohydrate	1g dietary fiber	0mg cholesterol	87mg sodium

2 large red bell peppers	½ tsp. ground black pepper
1 cup sun-dried tomatoes	½ tsp. crushed red pepper flakes
1 tsp. minced garlic	1 TB. lemon juice
1 TB. fresh thyme	2 TB. extra-virgin olive oil
1 TB. capers, drained	

1. Preheat a grill top or a grill to medium heat.

2. Place red bell peppers on the grill, and cook on all sides for about 20 minutes or until charred. Immediately place peppers on a plate, cover with plastic wrap, let cool for 10 minutes.

3. When peppers are cool enough to handle, peel off skin. (It's okay if it doesn't all come off.) Remove stalks and seeds.

4. In a food processor fitted with a chopping blade, pulse roasted red peppers and sun-dried tomatoes 10 times.

5. Add garlic, thyme, capers, black pepper, crushed red pepper flakes, lemon juice, and olive oil, and pulse 5 times.

6. Serve immediately, or refrigerate for up to 1 week.

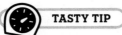 **TASTY TIP**

If you're using sun-dried tomatoes stored in olive oil, you can omit adding the extra-virgin olive oil in this recipe.

Baba Ganoush

Here, the smoky flavor of eggplant combines with fresh vegetables and olive oil. The result is light and refreshing.

Yield:	Prep time:	Cook time:	Serving size:
3 cups	20 minutes	50 minutes	2 tablespoons

Each serving has:			
36 calories	2g fat	0g saturated fat	1g protein
4g carbohydrate	2g dietary fiber	0mg cholesterol	99mg sodium

2 large eggplants

4 TB. extra-virgin olive oil

1 large white onion, chopped

1 TB. minced garlic

3 TB. fresh lemon juice

1 tsp. salt

$^1/_2$ tsp. ground black pepper

$^1/_2$ medium red bell pepper, ribs and seeds removed, and finely diced

$^1/_2$ medium green bell pepper, ribs and seeds removed, and finely diced

3 TB. fresh parsley, finely chopped

$^1/_2$ tsp. cayenne

3 medium radishes, finely diced

3 whole green onions, finely chopped

1. Preheat a grill top or a grill to medium-low heat.

2. Place eggplants on the grill, and roast on all sides for 40 minutes, turning every 5 minutes. Immediately place eggplants on a plate, cover with plastic wrap, let cool for 15 minutes.

3. Remove eggplant stems, and peel off as much skin as possible. (It's okay if it doesn't all come off.)

4. In a food processor fitted with a chopping blade, pulse eggplant 7 times. Transfer eggplant to a medium bowl.

5. In a medium saucepan over low heat, heat 2 tablespoons extra-virgin olive oil. Add white onion, and sauté, stirring occasionally, for 10 minutes. Add onions to eggplant.

6. Add garlic, lemon juice, salt, black pepper, red bell pepper, green bell pepper, and parsley to eggplant, and stir well.

7. Spread baba ganoush on a serving plate, and drizzle remaining 2 tablespoons extra-virgin olive oil over top. Sprinkle with cayenne, radishes, and green onions.

8. Serve cold or at room temperature.

Appealing Appetizers and Breads

The appetizers and breads in this chapter are full of flavor and will satisfy your predinner appetite or hold their own in any meal. If you like bread and butter, try the flavorful Rosemary Olive Bread with a good extra-virgin olive oil instead of butter.

A little planning can go a long way with appetizers. Many of these recipes can be made in advance, and you can just cook and serve when you're ready. I like to make the Cheese Rolls, Spinach Pies, and the Meat-Filled Phyllo recipes right up to the point of baking, but instead of cooking them, I put them on a baking sheet and freeze them. When they're frozen, I put them in an airtight bag or container and store them for a month or two. Then they're ready to go in the oven whenever I need a starter for a meal.

In This Chapter

- Amazing appetizers
- Quick and tasty bites
- Delicious breads

Hummus Appetizer Bites

These hummus bites are great as hors d'oeuvres for a party or a healthy snack before dinner. They deliver a mouthful of smooth and tangy hummus atop a flaky crust.

Yield:	Prep time:	Cook time:	Serving size:
12 bites	45 minutes	10 minutes	1 bite

Each serving has:			
229 calories	16g fat	5g saturated fat	5g protein
18g carbohydrate	2g dietary fiber	374mg cholesterol	13mg sodium

1¼ cups all-purpose flour	1 batch Traditional Hummus (recipe in Chapter 11)
½ tsp. salt	
5 TB. cold butter	1 tsp. paprika
2 TB. vegetable shortening	12 kalamata olives
¼ cup ice water	12 fresh parsley leaves

1. In a food processor fitted with a chopping blade, pulse 1 cup all-purpose flour and salt 5 times.

2. Add cold butter and vegetable shortening, and pulse for 1 minute or until mixture resembles coarse meal.

3. Continue to pulse while adding water for about 1 minute. Test dough; if it holds together when you pinch it, it doesn't require any additional moisture. If it does not come together, add another 3 tablespoons water.

4. Remove dough from the food processor, place in a plastic bag, form into a flat disc, and refrigerate for 30 minutes.

5. Preheat the oven to 425°F.

6. Remove dough from the plastic bag, and dust both sides with flour. Sprinkle your counter with flour.

7. Using a rolling pin, roll out dough to 1/4 inch thickness. Using a 2-inch circle cookie cutter, cut out 12 circles of dough. Gently mold dough circles into a mini muffin tin, and using a fork, gently poke dough.

8. Bake for 10 minutes. Remove from the oven, and set aside to cool.

9. Spoon about 1 tablespoon Traditional Hummus on top of each cooled piecrust, sprinkle with paprika, and top with 1 kalamata olive and 1 parsley leaf each. Serve immediately or refrigerate.

Aromatic Artichokes

Artichokes are native to the Mediterranean area. The earthy green flavor of the artichokes with the citrus garlic dressing in this recipe is refreshing and light.

Yield:	Prep time:	Cook time:	Serving size:
4 artichokes	15 minutes	45 minutes	1 artichoke

Each serving has:			
190 calories	14g fat	2g saturated fat	4g protein
16g carbohydrate	7g dietary fiber	0mg cholesterol	412mg sodium

4 artichokes	$^1/_3$ cup fresh lemon juice
6 cups water	$^1/_4$ cup extra-virgin olive oil
2 cloves garlic	$^1/_2$ tsp. salt
1 bay leaf	$^1/_2$ tsp. ground black pepper
2 tsp. minced garlic	

1. Using a pair of kitchen scissors, cut off the tips of artichoke leaves. With a sharp knife, cut 1 inch off top of artichokes. Pull off small leaves along base and stem, leaving only a 1-inch stem. Rinse artichokes in cold water.

2. In a steamer or large saucepan over medium-high heat, bring water, garlic cloves, and bay leaf to a simmer. Add steaming basket, place artichokes inside, cover, and steam for 40 minutes.

3. In a small bowl, whisk together minced garlic, lemon juice, extra-virgin olive oil, salt, and black pepper.

4. Transfer artichokes from the steamer to a serving dish, and spoon dressing over artichokes, being sure to get it between leaves.

5. Serve warm or cold.

 MEDITERRANEAN MORSEL

Ever eaten an artichoke? They might look complicated, but they're really easy. Simply peel off a leaf and place the white, fleshy part in your mouth. Using your teeth, pull off the pulp portion, and discard inedible part of the leaf.

Cheese Rolls

One bite of these Mediterranean cheese rolls, oozing cheese with fresh parsley and a crunchy outside, and you'll be hooked.

Yield:	Prep time:	Cook time:	Serving size:
20 rolls	25 minutes	5 minutes	1 roll

Each serving has:			
199 calories	9g fat	4g saturated fat	9g protein
19g carbohydrate	1g dietary fiber	35mg cholesterol	334mg sodium

1 cup ackawi cheese	1 large egg yolk, beaten
1 cup shredded mozzarella cheese	2 TB. water
2 TB. fresh parsley, finely chopped	1 pkg. egg roll dough (20 count)
1 large egg	4 TB. extra-virgin olive oil
$^1/_2$ tsp. ground black pepper	

1. In a large bowl, combine ackawi cheese, mozzarella cheese, parsley, egg, and black pepper.

2. In a small bowl, whisk together egg yolk and water.

3. Lay out 1 egg roll, place 2 tablespoons cheese mixture at one corner of egg roll, and brush opposite corner with egg yolk mixture.

4. Fold over side of egg roll, with cheese, to the middle. Fold in left and right sides, and complete rolling egg roll, using egg-brushed side to seal. Set aside, seal side down, and repeat with remaining egg rolls and cheese mixture.

5. In a skillet over low heat, heat 2 tablespoons extra-virgin olive oil. Add up to 4 cheese rolls, seal side down, and cook for 1 or 2 minutes per side or until browned. Repeat with remaining 2 tablespoons extra-virgin olive oil and egg rolls.

6. Serve warm.

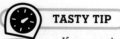 **TASTY TIP**

If you can't find ackawi cheese, don't fret. You can use any good melting cheese you like instead. Or you can use all mozzarella if you prefer.

Spinach Pies

These spinach pies have an earthy flavor with a hint of spice and a bright, citrus bite. They're great as a snack or even for lunch.

Yield:	Prep time:	Cook time:	Serving size:
18 pies	30 minutes	20 minutes	1 pie

Each serving has:			
189 calories	10g fat	1g saturated fat	4g protein
22g carbohydrate	2g dietary fiber	0mg cholesterol	271mg sodium

8 cups baby spinach, washed and chopped

1 tsp. salt

$1/4$ cup plus 4 TB. extra-virgin olive oil

1 large tomato, finely diced

1 large yellow onion, finely chopped

$1/4$ cup fresh lemon juice

$1/4$ tsp. cayenne

1 tsp. sumac

1 batch Multipurpose Dough (recipe later in this chapter)

1. In a large bowl, combine spinach and salt. Set aside for 20 minutes.

2. Preheat the oven to 400°F. Grease a baking sheet with 2 tablespoons extra-virgin olive oil.

3. Drain spinach and squeeze to remove any excess liquid. Place spinach in a separate large bowl.

4. Add tomato, yellow onion, lemon juice, $1/4$ cup extra-virgin olive oil, cayenne, and sumac to spinach, and mix well.

5. Dust a rolling pin and counter with all-purpose flour, and roll out 18 Multipurpose Dough balls to 5-inch discs $1/4$ inch thick.

6. Add 2 tablespoons spinach mixture to center of dough discs. Fold over and pinch together top portion halfway down. Bring up the bottom half, and pinch to top two halves. This should form a triangle.

7. Place spinach pies on the prepared baking sheet. Brush top of pies with remaining 2 tablespoons extra-virgin olive oil.

8. Bake for 18 to 20 minutes or until lightly browned.

9. Serve warm or cold.

Meat-Filled Phyllo (*Samboosek*)

These flaky little phyllo pies are full of seasoned beef. As a bonus, as the buttery toasted phyllo dough bakes, it will fill your house with an amazing aroma.

Yield:	Prep time:	Cook time:	Serving size:
12 phyllo pies	20 minutes	10 minutes	1 phyllo pie

Each serving has:			
321 calories	22g fat	12g saturated fat	10g protein
21g carbohydrate	1g dietary fiber	63mg cholesterol	508mg sodium

1 lb. ground beef or lamb	1 tsp. salt
1 medium yellow onion, finely chopped	1 pkg. frozen phyllo dough (12 sheets)
1 TB. seven spices	$^2/_3$ cup butter, melted

1. In a medium skillet over medium heat, brown beef for 3 minutes, breaking up chunks with a wooden spoon.

2. Add yellow onion, seven spices, and salt, and cook for 5 to 7 minutes or until beef is browned and onions are translucent. Set aside, and let cool.

3. Place first sheet of phyllo on your work surface, brush with melted butter, lay second sheet of phyllo on top, and brush with melted butter. Cut sheets into 3-inch-wide strips.

4. Spoon 2 tablespoons meat filling at end of each strip, and fold end strip to cover meat and form a triangle. Fold pointed end up and over to the opposite end, and you should see a triangle forming. Continue to fold up and then over until you come to the end of strip.

5. Place phyllo pies on a baking sheet, seal side down, and brush tops with butter. Repeat with remaining phyllo and filling.

6. Bake for 10 minutes or until golden brown.

7. Remove from the oven and set aside for 5 minutes before serving warm or at room temperature.

 MEDITERRANEAN MORSEL

Phyllo dough is very flaky and dries out very fast, so you have to work quickly when using it. Keep the unused phyllo covered with a damp cloth or sealed in a plastic bag until you're ready for it.

Beef Tartar (*Kibbeh Nayeh*)

Kibbeh Nayeh is raw, spiced beef mixed with bulgur wheat and eaten smeared on pita bread with veggies and extra-virgin olive oil.

Yield:	Prep time:	Serving size:	
2$^1/_2$ cups	45 minutes	2 tablespoons	
Each serving has:			
55 calories	4g fat	1g saturated fat	2g protein
2g carbohydrate	1g dietary fiber	7mg cholesterol	124mg sodium

$^1/_2$ cup bulgur wheat, grind #1

1 cup warm water

$^1/_4$ cup toasted walnuts

3 fresh basil leaves

2 TB. fresh parsley, chopped

$^1/_2$ medium white onion, chopped

$^1/_2$ large red bell pepper, ribs and seeds removed, and roughly chopped

1 tsp. crushed red pepper flakes

1 tsp. paprika

1 tsp. salt

$^1/_2$ tsp. ground black pepper

$^1/_4$ tsp. ground cloves

$^1/_4$ tsp. cumin

$^1/_4$ tsp. ground cinnamon

$^1/_2$ tsp. dried ground sage

$^1/_4$ tsp. ground allspice

$^1/_4$ tsp. ground nutmeg

$^1/_4$ tsp. ground coriander

$^1/_2$ lb. lean ground chuck beef

3 TB. extra-virgin olive oil

1. In a medium bowl, combine bulgur wheat and warm water. Set aside for 30 minutes.

2. In a food processor fitted with a chopping blade, blend bulgur, walnuts, basil, parsley, white onion, and red bell pepper for 1 minute.

3. Add crushed red pepper flakes, paprika, salt, black pepper, cloves, cumin, cinnamon, sage, allspice, nutmeg, and coriander, and blend for 30 seconds.

4. Add ground chuck, and blend for 1 minute.

5. Spread meat mixture on a plate, drizzle extra-virgin olive oil on top, and serve with pita bread and fresh vegetables.

 MEDITERRANEAN MORSEL

There are always concerns when eating any raw meat, especially for children or elderly. Do your due diligence before eating any raw meat.

Pita Bread

This soft, chewy flatbread is perfect for rolling into a sandwich or using as a pocket and stuffing with your favorite sandwich filling.

Yield:	Prep time:	Cook time:	Serving size:
10 pitas	$2^1/_2$ hours	10 minutes	1 pita

Each serving has:			
205 calories	6g fat	1g saturated fat	5g protein
32g carbohydrate	2g dietary fiber	0mg cholesterol	234mg sodium

$1^1/_2$ TB. active dry yeast	4 TB. extra-virgin olive oil
$1^1/_2$ cups warm water	1 tsp. salt
1 tsp. sugar	3 cups all-purpose flour

1. In a large bowl, combine yeast, warm water, and sugar, and set aside for 5 minutes.

2. Add 3 tablespoons extra-virgin olive oil, salt, and 1 cup all-purpose flour, and stir to combine. Add another 1 cup all-purpose flour, and begin to knead dough. Add remaining 1 cup all-purpose flour, and knead for about 3 minutes or until dough comes together in a ball. If you're using an electric stand mixer, use the dough attachment to knead dough.

3. Remove dough from the bowl, and grease the bowl with remaining 1 tablespoon extra-virgin olive oil. Return dough to the bowl, and turn over to coat dough in oil. Cover the bowl with plastic wrap and a thick towel, and set aside to rise for 2 hours.

4. Preheat the oven to 475°F.

5. Uncover the bowl, and gently pull dough together into a ball. Divide dough into 10 equal-size pieces, lightly dust with flour, and cover with plastic wrap or a moist towel.

6. Flour your rolling pin and work surface. Roll out each dough ball to $^1/_4$ inch thick, and place on a baking sheet. Let rolled-out dough sit for 10 minutes before baking.

7. Bake for 3 or 4 minutes or just until dough puffs up into a ball. Remove from the oven, and using a spatula, transfer pitas onto a plate and cover with a lightly dampened towel. (If a pita pocket does not form when baked, spritz the next batch with some water and continue to bake.)

8. Store pitas in a bag, and enjoy for up to 1 week.

MEDITERRANEAN MORSEL

Instead of baking it, you can cook the pita dough on a stovetop. Preheat an iron or cast-iron skillet over medium-low heat, and brush lightly with extra-virgin olive oil. Add 1 rolled-out dough to the skillet, and cook for 2 or 3 minutes or until lightly browned. Flip over and cook for 2 more minutes. Transfer to a plate, and cover with a slightly damp towel. Brush the skillet with more extra-virgin olive oil before cooking the next pita.

Savory Pita Chips

I love pita chips. They quench the craving for crunch without the guilt of a bag of potato chips. I also love these seasoned pita chips because they deliver a touch of extra flavor.

Yield:	Prep time:	Cook time:	Serving size:
6 cups	10 minutes	10 minutes	1 cup
Each serving has:			
201 calories	11g fat	2g saturated fat	4g protein
23g carbohydrate	4g dietary fiber	0mg cholesterol	554mg sodium

3 pitas	$^1/_4$ cup zaatar
$^1/_4$ cup extra-virgin olive oil	

1. Preheat the oven to 450°F.

2. Cut pitas into 2-inch pieces, and place in a large bowl.

3. Drizzle pitas with extra-virgin olive oil, sprinkle with zaatar, and toss to coat.

4. Spread out pitas on a baking sheet, and bake for 8 to 10 minutes or until lightly browned and crunchy.

5. Let pita chips cool before removing from the baking sheet. Store in an airtight container for up to 1 month.

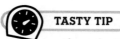 **TASTY TIP**

If you don't like or don't have zaatar spice, you can instead use a combination of your favorite ground herbs or spices to season your pita chips.

Rosemary Olive Bread

This seasoned herb bread is light, flavorful, and very versatile. I love to make batches of it, freeze it, and bake some when I have the craving!

Yield:	Prep time:	Cook time:	Serving size:
10 pitas	2¹/₂ hours	20 minutes	1 pita

Each serving has:			
254 calories	11g fat	1g saturated fat	5g protein
33g carbohydrate	2g dietary fiber	0mg cholesterol	292mg sodium

1¹/₂ TB. active dry yeast

1¹/₂ cups warm water

1 tsp. sugar

1 tsp. salt

¹/₄ cup plus 3 TB. extra-virgin olive oil

3 TB. fresh rosemary, roughly chopped

10 kalamata olives, pitted and roughly chopped

1 tsp. ground black pepper

3 cups all-purpose flour

1. In a large bowl, combine yeast, warm water, and sugar, and set aside for 5 minutes.

2. Add salt, ¹/₄ cup extra-virgin olive oil, rosemary, kalamata olives, black pepper, and 1 cup all-purpose flour, and stir to combine. Add another 1 cup all-purpose flour, and begin to knead dough. Add remaining 1 cup all-purpose flour, and knead for about 3 minutes or until dough comes together in a ball. If you're using an electric stand mixer, use the dough attachment to knead dough.

3. Remove dough from the bowl, and grease the bowl with 1 tablespoon extra-virgin olive oil. Return dough to the bowl, and turn over to coat dough in oil. Cover the bowl with plastic wrap and a thick towel, and set aside to rise for 2 hours.

4. Uncover the bowl, and gently pull dough together into a ball. Divide dough into 10 equal-size pieces, lightly dust with flour and cover with plastic wrap or a moist towel.

5. Flour your rolling pin and work surface. Roll out each dough ball to ¹/₄ inch thick, and place on a baking sheet. Let rolled-out dough sit for 10 minutes before cooking.

6. Preheat an iron or cast-iron skillet over medium-low heat, and brush lightly with extra-virgin olive oil. Add 1 rolled-out dough to the skillet, and cook for 2 or 3 minutes or until lightly browned. Flip over and cook for 2 more minutes. Transfer to a plate, and cover with a slightly damp towel. Brush the skillet with more extra-virgin olive oil before cooking next piece.

7. Store in an airtight container, and serve with a good extra-virgin olive oil and olives.

Multipurpose Dough

This tender and flaky dough is so versatile, you can use it to make pita bread, pizza, spinach pies, or rolls—which is what this recipe offers instructions for.

Yield:	Prep time:	Cook time:	Serving size:
16 rolls	$2^1/_2$ hours	20 minutes	1 roll
Each serving has:			
114 calories	3g fat	0g saturated fat	3g protein
18g carbohydrate	1g dietary fiber	0mg cholesterol	130mg sodium

$1^1/_2$ TB. active dry yeast	1 tsp. salt
$1^1/_2$ cups warm water	3 cups all-purpose flour
1 tsp. sugar	2 TB. cornmeal
6 TB. extra-virgin olive oil	

1. In a large bowl, combine yeast, warm water, and sugar, and set aside for 5 minutes.

2. Add 3 tablespoons extra-virgin olive oil, salt, and 1 cup all-purpose flour, and stir to combine. Add another 1 cup all-purpose flour, and begin to knead dough. Add remaining 1 cup all-purpose flour, and knead for about 3 minutes or until dough comes together in a ball. If you're using an electric stand mixer, use the dough attachment to knead dough.

3. Remove dough from the bowl, and grease the bowl with 1 tablespoon extra-virgin olive oil. Return dough to the bowl, and turn over to coat dough in oil. Cover the bowl with plastic wrap and a thick towel, and set aside to rise for 2 hours.

4. Preheat the oven to 420°F. Dust a baking sheet with cornmeal.

5. Uncover the bowl, and gently pull dough together into a ball. Divide dough into 16 pieces, lightly dust with flour, and place on the baking sheet about 2 inches apart. Bake for 20 minutes or until golden brown.

6. Transfer rolls to a plate, and brush with remaining 2 tablespoons extra-virgin olive oil.

7. Serve immediately or store in an airtight container.

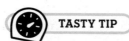 **TASTY TIP**

If you're not going to be using the dough for rolls or any other item right away, you can store the dough in a plastic container or bag for up to 2 months in the freezer.

Sauces, Spices, and Condiments

The nice thing about the Mediterranean diet is that you can add tons of flavor without a lot of fat, thanks to sauces, seasoning blends, and condiments in this chapter.

Instead of spreading butter on your toasted bread, try some Lemon Basil Garlic Sauce and make your own garlic bread. Instead of buying your morning yogurt, try making a nice big batch of Homemade Greek Yogurt. Scoop a cup full for breakfast and add whatever fresh fruit or oats you'd like, and you have a fresh breakfast that's low in sugar. Familiarizing yourself with these basic recipes can help you liven any plate.

Spices and herbs add an abundance of flavor with minimal calories. Use herbs fresh or dried—each adds a different flavor. And don't skimp on the spices. There are so many to choose from; experiment to determine what you like. Two common spices used in many Mediterranean countries are Zaatar and Seven Spice Mix. Zaatar, which is a blend of dried thyme and sumac, is used to season salads, breads, and so much more. Seven Spice Mix's earthy flavor goes with any protein.

In This Chapter

- Sensational sauces
- Getting spicy
- Condiments you'll crave

Tzatziki Sauce

This yogurt-cucumber sauce has a cool and refreshing flavor, thanks to the tangy Greek yogurt and the refreshing mint. It's a great accompaniment to any spicy dish.

Yield:	Prep time:	Serving size:	
4 cups	5 minutes	$^1/_2$ cup	

Each serving has:			
37 calories	0g fat	0g saturated fat	5g protein
4g carbohydrate	1g dietary fiber	2mg cholesterol	162mg sodium

2 cups plain Greek yogurt

3 medium Persian cucumbers, finely diced

2 TB. fresh lemon juice

1 TB. minced garlic

$^1/_2$ tsp. salt

1 tsp. dried mint

$^1/_2$ cup water

1. In a large bowl, combine Greek yogurt, Persian cucumbers, lemon juice, garlic, salt, mint, and water, and stir for about 15 seconds.

2. Serve immediately, or refrigerate in an airtight container for up to 3 days.

 TASTY TIP

Many regions make tzatziki sauce slightly different. The Greek use fresh dill, while the Lebanese use dried mint. You can use either one, depending on what flavor you like. If you want to use dill, replace the dried mint called for with 1 tablespoon chopped fresh dill.

Homemade Greek Yogurt

I love the tangy flavor of Greek yogurt! When I was a kid, my mom would make us eat a bowl of it after we'd played outside all day. She said it would cool us down—and it did. This cool, smooth, and tangy yogurt is so tasty.

Yield:	Prep time:	Cook time:	Serving size:
12 cups	2 days	20 minutes	$1/_2$ cup

Each serving has:			
111 calories	5g fat	3g saturated fat	7g protein
8g carbohydrate	0g dietary fiber	23mg cholesterol	93mg sodium

1 gal. whole milk	2 cups plain Greek yogurt

1. In a large pot over medium-low heat, bring whole milk to a simmer until a froth starts to form on the surface. If you have a thermometer, bring the milk to 185°F.

2. Remove from heat, and let milk cool to lukewarm, or 110°F.

3. Pour all but about 2 cups milk into a large plastic container.

4. Pour remaining 2 cups milk into a smaller bowl. Add Greek yogurt, and stir until well combined.

5. Slowly pour milk and yogurt mixture into the large bowl of milk, and stir well.

6. Cover the bowl with a lid, and set aside where it won't be disturbed. Cover it with a towel, and let it sit overnight.

7. The next morning, gently transfer the bowl to the refrigerator. Chill for at least 1 day.

8. The next day, gently pour off clear liquid that's formed on top of yogurt, leaving just a little liquid remaining.

9. Serve, or store in the refrigerator for up to 2 weeks.

 MEDITERRANEAN MORSEL

When your yogurt is complete, take out 2 cups to save it as a starter for your next batch. My mom would always forget and send me to my aunt's house to pick up some starter.

Tahini Paste

Tahini paste isn't meant to be eaten raw. It has a toasted, bitter flavor. Instead, use it to make a sauce, dressing, or—better yet—hummus, and you'll have an amazing recipe.

Yield:	Prep time:	Cook time:	Serving size:
2 cups	10 minutes	4 minutes	2 tablespoons

Each serving has:			
148 calories	15g fat	2g saturated fat	4g protein
2g carbohydrate	2g dietary fiber	0mg cholesterol	9mg sodium

2 cups hulled sesame seeds	¼ cup vegetable oil

1. Preheat the oven to 450°F.

2. Evenly spread sesame seeds on a baking sheet, and toast in the oven for 4 minutes.

3. Remove from the oven, and carefully add sesame seeds to a food processor fitted with a chopping blade. Add vegetable oil, and blend for 2 minutes.

4. Stop the food processor, and scrape down the sides of the bowl with a rubber spatula. Blend for 2 more minutes. Repeat one more time until you have a smooth texture.

5. Store in a sealed glass jar in the pantry for up to 3 months.

 MEDITERRANEAN MORSEL

Sometimes, if a jar of tahini paste sits for a long period of time, a layer of oil forms on the top. This is just the oil separating from the rest of the particles and rising to the top. The tahini is still good. Just shake the jar or stir it before using.

Tahini Sauce (*Tarator*)

This dipping sauce is great for falafel or as a dressing for a salad. Tahini sauce has a nutty flavor followed by a bit of tang, thanks to lemon juice and a hint of garlic.

Yield:	Prep time:	Serving size:	
2 cups	5 minutes	2 tablespoons	
Each serving has:			
76 calories	7g fat	1g saturated fat	2g protein
2g carbohydrate	1g dietary fiber	0mg cholesterol	78mg sodium

1 cup Tahini Paste (recipe earlier in this chapter)

$^1/_3$ cup lemon juice

1 TB. minced garlic

$^2/_3$ cup water

$^1/_2$ tsp. salt

1 TB. fresh parsley, chopped

1 TB. fresh chopped radish

1. In a large bowl, whisk together Tahini Paste, lemon juice, garlic, water, and salt.

2. Store in an airtight container in the refrigerator for up to 1 week. When ready to serve, top with a sprinkle of parsley and chopped radish.

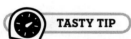 **TASTY TIP**

If you like your sauce thicker, reduce the amount of water. If you like your sauce thinner, add a bit more water.

Garlic Sauce

This sauce is the perfect condiment for pretty much anything if you love garlic. The creamy, smooth, mayonnaise-type sauce has a little bit of tang from the lemon and a whole lot of bold garlic flavor.

Yield:	Prep time:	Serving size:	
4 cups	10 minutes	1 tablespoon	
Each serving has:			
94 calories	10g fat	1g saturated fat	0g protein
1g carbohydrate	0g dietary fiber	0mg cholesterol	37mg sodium

1 cup garlic cloves	¹/₂ cup fresh lemon juice
1 tsp. salt	3 cups canola oil

1. In a food processor fitted with a chopping blade, blend garlic and salt for 30 seconds. Stop the food processor, and scrape down the sides of the bowl with a rubber spatula. Replace the lid.

2. Turn the food processor back on, and pour in 2 tablespoons lemon juice through the top hole. Slowly drizzle in ¹/₃ cup canola oil, and blend for 30 seconds. Stop the food processor, and scrape down the sides again.

3. Turn the food processor back on, and continue to very slowly add remaining lemon juice and canola oil—alternating as you go. This should take about 3 to 5 minutes, and a thick, mayonnaise-type sauce should form.

4. Store in a sealed glass jar in the refrigerator for up to 3 months.

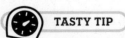 **TASTY TIP**

This sauce makes a great dip for chicken or french fries, or spread on a sandwich. I even spread it on a loaf of bread and top with some cheese to make garlic bread. You can use it as a marinade for grilled chicken or steak, too.

Lemon Basil Garlic Sauce

This sauce is an amazing fusion of fresh basil and pungent garlic with the zestiness of lemon. It brightens the flavor of almost anything it's served with.

Yield:	Prep time:	Serving size:	
4 cups	10 minutes	1 tablespoon	
Each serving has:			
94 calories	10g fat	1g saturated fat	0g protein
1g carbohydrate	0g dietary fiber	0mg cholesterol	37mg sodium

1 cup garlic cloves

1 tsp. salt

$^1/_2$ cup fresh lemon juice

3 cups canola oil

$^1/_4$ cup fresh basil, chopped

1 TB. lemon zest

$^1/_2$ tsp. ground black pepper

1. In a food processor fitted with a chopping blade, blend garlic and salt for 30 seconds. Stop the food processor, and scrape down the sides of the bowl with a rubber spatula. Replace the lid.

2. Turn the food processor back on, pour in 2 tablespoons lemon juice, slowly drizzle in $^1/_3$ cup canola oil, and blend for 30 seconds. Stop the food processor, and scrape down the sides again.

3. Turn the food processor back on, and continue to very slowly add remaining lemon juice and canola oil—alternating as you go. This should take about 3 to 5 minutes, and a thick, mayonnaise-type sauce should form.

4. Add basil, lemon zest, and black pepper to the food processor, and pulse for 30 seconds.

5. Store in a sealed glass jar in the refrigerator for up to 1 month.

Hot Sauce (*Harissa*)

Harissa is a spicy but flavorful hot sauce that combines dried chiles with a hint of garlic and olive tones from the extra-virgin olive oil.

Yield:	Prep time:	Serving size:	
1 cup	45 minutes	1 teaspoon	
Each serving has:			
21 calories	2g fat	0g saturated fat	0g protein
0g carbohydrate	0g dietary fiber	0mg cholesterol	25mg sodium

20 dried red chili (cayenne) peppers	$^1/_2$ tsp. ground coriander seeds
2 cups hot water	$^1/_2$ tsp. caraway seeds
3 cloves garlic	$^1/_2$ tsp. cumin
$^1/_2$ tsp. salt	$^1/_2$ cup extra-virgin olive oil

1. Place red chili peppers in a medium bowl, pour hot water over top, and set aside to soak for 30 minutes.

2. Drain hot water, and remove stems and seeds from peppers. It's recommended that you wear latex gloves while doing this.

3. In a food processor fitted with a chopping blade, blend red chili peppers, garlic, salt, coriander, caraway seeds, and cumin for 2 minutes.

4. With the food processor still running, drizzle in extra-virgin olive oil, and blend for 30 more seconds.

5. Store in a sealed glass jar in the refrigerator for up to 1 month.

Zaatar

This spice mix is very earthy. The thyme lends a bright, earthy flavor while the sumac provides a slight tang.

Yield:	Prep time:	Cook time:	Serving size:
1 cup	5 minutes	3 minutes	1 tablespoon

Each serving has:			
15 calories	1g fat	0g saturated fat	0g protein
2g carbohydrate	1g dietary fiber	0mg cholesterol	148mg sodium

2 TB. sesame seeds	2 TB. sumac, ground
³/₄ cup dried thyme, ground	1 tsp. salt

1. Preheat the oven to 400°F.

2. Spread sesame seeds on a baking sheet, and toast for 3 minutes. Remove toasted seeds from the baking sheet, and set aside to cool.

3. In a small bowl, combine thyme, sumac, sesame seeds, and salt.

4. Store in an airtight container.

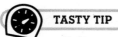 **TASTY TIP**

Zaatar is a very versatile spice blend. You can mix it with olive oil and use it as a dip for fresh bread. Or spread it on rolled dough and bake into a breakfast pizza called *manoushi*. Or sprinkle it on Yogurt Spread (*Labne;* recipe in Chapter 3) or a salad for a tangy twist.

Seven Spice Mix

This is my go-to spice mix. It's used very often in Mediterranean cooking and gives food a sweet and spicy flavor with a hint of smokiness from the allspice.

Yield:	Prep time:	Serving size:	
7 tablespoons	5 minutes	1 tablespoon	
Each serving has:			
24 calories	1g fat	0g saturated fat	1g protein
5g carbohydrate	3g dietary fiber	0mg cholesterol	5mg sodium

1 TB. ground black pepper

1 TB. ground allspice

1 TB. ground cinnamon

1 TB. ground nutmeg

1 TB. ground coriander

1 TB. ground cloves

1 TB. ground ginger

1. In a glass jar with a lid, add black pepper, allspice, cinnamon, nutmeg, coriander, cloves, and ginger. Apply the lid, and shake to combine.

2. Store in a dry place for up to 6 months.

Mouthwatering Mediterranean Mains

Mediterranean main dishes are all about satisfaction, prepared with tantalizing herbs and spices and rich and flavorful proteins, vegetables, and grains. In Part 5, I give you some recipes that are quick and easy to prepare but bursting with flavor, and some others that take a little more time and care.

From meaty morsels to versatile veggie-based main dishes to sides that could almost steal the show, you're sure to discover new Mediterranean-based favorites in the following chapters.

Beef and Lamb Dinners

Many Mediterranean main dishes focus on a protein as the main ingredient, whether that protein is chicken, beef, lamb, shrimp, fish, or beans. The great thing is that you can interchange many of the proteins to suit your taste. In this chapter, the recipes focus on lean red meats.

In the Mediterranean diet guidelines, it's important to get the protein and iron red meat contains but still eat it sparingly because it can be high in saturated fat. Limiting your intake to four or fives times a month is key.

In addition, learning what cut to buy can be helpful. When a recipe calls for ground beef or lamb, choose a blend of 95/5, which is only 5 percent fat. If you're craving a steak, opt for the fillet cut, which has very minimal fat and a lot of flavor.

In This Chapter

- Beefy main dishes
- Lamb entrées
- Filling pockets and pies
- Choosing your cut

Beef Shawarma

This beef dish is marinated in an abundance of spices, with a hint of citrus and flavorful garlic. Shawarma meat makes the best sandwiches.

Yield:	Prep time:	Cook time:	Serving size:
1 pound steak	30 minutes	20 minutes	¹/₄ pound

Each serving has:			
358 calories	24g fat	7g saturated fat	30g protein
4g carbohydrate	1g dietary fiber	68mg cholesterol	669mg sodium

1 lb. skirt steak	1 tsp. salt
2 TB. minced garlic	¹/₂ tsp. ground black pepper
¹/₄ cup fresh lemon juice	¹/₄ tsp. ground cinnamon
2 TB. apple cider vinegar	¹/₄ tsp. ground cardamom
3 TB. extra-virgin olive oil	1 tsp. seven spices

1. Using a sharp knife, cut skirt steak into thin, ¹/₄-inch strips. Place strips in a large bowl.

2. Add garlic, lemon juice, apple cider vinegar, extra-virgin olive oil, salt, black pepper, cinnamon, cardamom, and seven spices, and mix well.

3. Place steak in the refrigerator and marinate for at least 20 minutes and up to 24 hours.

4. Preheat a large skillet over medium heat. Add meat and marinade, and cook for 20 minutes or until meat is tender and marinade has evaporated.

5. Serve warm with pita bread and tahini sauce.

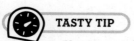 **TASTY TIP**

You can switch out the beef for lamb in this recipe and have a wonderful dish.

Kefta Kabob

This is a very popular dish all along the Mediterranean region, and it's basically the same recipe anywhere you go. Ground meat is seasoned with some light spices and then grilled to perfection.

Yield:	Prep time:	Cook time:	Serving size:
4 kabobs	10 minutes	7 minutes	1 kabob

Each serving has:			
276 calories	18g fat	7g saturated fat	25g protein
3g carbohydrate	1g dietary fiber	88mg cholesterol	669mg sodium

$^1/_2$ large yellow onion, chopped	1 tsp. salt
$^1/_2$ cup fresh Italian parsley	$^1/_2$ tsp. ground black pepper
$^3/_4$ lb. ground beef	$^1/_2$ tsp. ground nutmeg
$^1/_4$ lb. ground lamb	$^1/_2$ tsp. seven spices

1. Preheat a grill to medium heat.

2. In a food processor fitted with a chopping blade, pulse yellow onion and Italian parsley for 30 seconds.

3. In a medium bowl, combine onion-parsley mixture, beef, lamb, salt, black pepper, nutmeg, and seven spices. Form mixture into 4 (6-inch) kabobs.

4. Grill kabobs, turning them over every 2 minutes, to cook on all sides.

5. Serve warm with hummus and pita bread.

 TASTY TIP

Many people don't like lamb. If you don't like it, you can omit the lamb and use 1 pound ground beef instead. (Although in this recipe, you really can't taste the lamb; it makes the kabob juicier.)

Kibbeh with Yogurt

In this dish, full of fiber and protein, ground beef is combined with earthy bulgur wheat and spices and cooked in a warm yogurt sauce.

Yield:	Prep time:	Cook time:	Serving size:
12 kibbeh	45 minutes	50 minutes	1 kibbeh

Each serving has:			
236 calories	14g fat	3g saturated fat	19g protein
8g carbohydrate	1g dietary fiber	37mg cholesterol	451mg sodium

$^1/_2$ cup bulgur wheat, grind #1

4 cups water

1 large yellow onion, chopped

2 fresh basil leaves

1 lb. lean ground chuck beef

2 tsp. salt

1 tsp. ground black pepper

$^1/_2$ tsp. ground allspice

$^1/_2$ tsp. ground coriander

$^1/_2$ tsp. ground cumin

$^1/_2$ tsp. ground nutmeg

$^1/_2$ tsp. ground cloves

$^1/_2$ tsp. ground cinnamon

$^1/_2$ tsp. dried sage

$^1/_4$ cup long-grain rice

$^1/_2$ lb. ground beef

3 TB. extra-virgin olive oil

$^1/_2$ cup pine nuts

1 tsp. seven spices

4 cups Greek yogurt

2 TB. minced garlic

1 tsp. dried mint

1. In a small bowl, soak bulgur wheat in 1 cup water for 30 minutes.

2. In a food processor fitted with a chopping blade, blend $^1/_2$ of yellow onion and basil for 30 seconds. Add bulgur, and blend for 30 more seconds.

3. Add ground chuck, $1^1/_2$ teaspoons salt, black pepper, allspice, coriander, cumin, nutmeg, cloves, cinnamon, and sage, and blend for 1 minute.

4. Transfer mixture to a large bowl, and knead for 3 minutes.

5. In a large pot, combine long-grain rice and remaining 3 cups water, and cook for 30 minutes.

6. In a medium skillet over medium heat, brown beef for 5 minutes, breaking up chunks with a wooden spoon.

7. Add remaining $^1/_2$ of yellow onion, extra-virgin olive oil, remaining $^1/_2$ teaspoon salt, pine nuts, and seven spices, and cook for 7 minutes. Set aside to cool.

8. Whisk Greek yogurt into cooked rice, add garlic and mint, reduce heat to low, and cook for 5 minutes.

9. Form meat-bulgur mixture into 12 equal-size balls. Create a groove in center of each ball, fill with beef and onion mixture, and seal groove.

10. Carefully drop balls into yogurt sauce, and cook for 15 minutes. Serve warm.

Kibbeh in a Pan

This version of kibbeh is prepared a bit differently from the preceding recipe. Here, ground meat is combined with earthy bulgur wheat and spices, layered in a baking dish, and baked until golden brown.

Yield:	Prep time:	Cook time:	Serving size:
12 kibbeh	55 minutes	37 minutes	1 kibbeh

Each serving has:			
215 calories	17g fat	4g saturated fat	11g protein
4g carbohydrate	1g dietary fiber	33mg cholesterol	423mg sodium

$^1/_2$ cup bulgur wheat, grind #1	$^1/_2$ tsp. ground cumin
1 cup water	$^1/_2$ tsp. ground nutmeg
1 large yellow onion, chopped	$^1/_2$ tsp. ground cloves
2 fresh basil leaves	$^1/_2$ tsp. ground cinnamon
1 lb. lean ground chuck beef	$^1/_2$ tsp. dried sage
2 tsp. salt	$^1/_2$ lb. ground beef
1 tsp. ground black pepper	4 TB. extra-virgin olive oil
$^1/_2$ tsp. ground allspice	$^1/_2$ cup pine nuts
$^1/_2$ tsp. ground coriander	1 tsp. seven spices

1. In a small bowl, soak bulgur wheat in water for 30 minutes.

2. In a food processor fitted with a chopping blade, blend $^1/_2$ of yellow onion and basil for 30 seconds. Add bulgur, and blend for 30 more seconds.

3. Add ground chuck, $1^1/_2$ teaspoons salt, black pepper, allspice, coriander, cumin, nutmeg, cloves, cinnamon, and sage, and blend for 1 minute.

4. Transfer mixture to a large bowl, and knead for 3 minutes.

5. In a medium skillet over medium heat, brown beef for 5 minutes, breaking up chunks with a wooden spoon.

6. Add remaining $^1/_2$ of yellow onion, 2 tablespoons extra-virgin olive oil, remaining $^1/_2$ teaspoon salt, pine nuts, and seven spices, and cook for 7 minutes.

7. Preheat the oven to 450°F. Grease an 8×8-inch baking dish with extra-virgin olive oil.

8. Divide kibbeh dough in half, spread a layer of dough on bottom of the prepared baking dish, add a layer of sautéed vegetables, and top with remaining kibbeh dough.

9. Paint top of kibbeh with remaining 2 tablespoons extra-virgin olive oil, and cut kibbeh into 12 equal-size pieces. Bake for 25 minutes.

10. Let kibbeh rest for 15 minutes before serving.

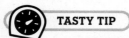 **TASTY TIP**

You also can fry kibbeh. Form the dough into balls, and stuff with the filling. Fry the kibbeh in a pan with vegetable oil for 6 minutes, and drain on a plate lined with paper towels.

Beef Shish Kabobs

Here, tender pieces of juicy fillet are seasoned with a hint of spice and smoky vegetables and cooked to your liking.

Yield:	Prep time:	Cook time:	Serving size:
5 kabobs	15 minutes	6 minutes	1 kabob
Each serving has:			
205 calories	7g fat	3g saturated fat	27g protein
7g carbohydrate	2g dietary fiber	72mg cholesterol	523mg sodium

1 lb. beef fillet	1 tsp. seven spices
1 large green bell pepper, seeds and ribs removed	1 tsp. salt
1 large white onion, peeled	1 tsp. ground black pepper
	3 TB. extra-virgin olive oil

1. Preheat a grill to medium heat.

2. Cut beef fillet into $^3/_4$-inch cubes, and place in a large bowl.

3. Cut green bell pepper into $^3/_4$-inch pieces. Cut white onion into 8 sections, and separate layers. Add bell pepper and onion to beef fillet.

4. Add seven spices, salt, black pepper, and extra-virgin olive oil, and mix to coat all ingredients evenly.

5. Skewer meat, onions, and bell pepper, alternating each on the skewer until you have 5 equal-size skewers.

6. Place the skewers on the grill. For medium-cooked meat, grill for a total of 10 minutes, rotating skewers every 2 minutes, or until evenly grilled on all sides. Serve warm.

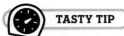 **TASTY TIP**

If you like more grilled vegetables with your meat, try adding some crimini mushrooms, zucchini, or cherry tomatoes to your beef skewers.

Tomato and Beef Casserole

This casserole is full of happy flavors. Seasoned beef is baked and topped with potato slices and a seasoned tomato sauce. It gives you protein, potassium, and carotenoids, all in one dish.

Yield:	Prep time:	Cook time:	Serving size:
1 (8×8-inch) casserole	20 minutes	55 minutes	$^1/_6$ of casserole

Each serving has:			
376 calories	16g fat	4g saturated fat	18g protein
39g carbohydrate	4g dietary fiber	44mg cholesterol	1,057mg sodium

$^1/_2$ medium yellow onion, chopped	3 TB. extra-virgin olive oil
1 lb. ground beef	1 (16-oz.) can plain tomato sauce
2 tsp. salt	1 cup water
1 tsp. ground black pepper	$^1/_2$ tsp. garlic powder
8 small red potatoes, washed and scrubbed	$^1/_2$ tsp. dried oregano

1. Preheat the oven to 450°F.

2. In a food processor fitted with a chopping blade, blend yellow onion for 30 seconds.

3. In a large bowl, combine onions, beef, 1 teaspoon salt, and $^1/_2$ teaspoon black pepper.

4. Spread beef mixture in an even layer in the bottom of a deep, 8×8-inch casserole dish. Bake for 20 minutes.

5. Slice red potatoes into $1/4$-inch slices, and place in a bowl. Drizzle extra-virgin olive oil over top, and toss to coat. Evenly spread out potatoes on a baking sheet, and bake for 20 minutes.

6. In a medium saucepan over low heat, combine tomato sauce, water, remaining 1 teaspoon salt, remaining $1/2$ teaspoon black pepper, garlic powder, and oregano. Cook for 10 minutes.

7. Remove casserole and potatoes from the oven, and using a spatula, spoon potatoes over beef. Pour tomato sauce over beef and potatoes, and bake for 15 minutes.

8. Serve warm with brown rice.

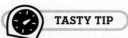 **TASTY TIP**

   If you like tomatoes, add a layer of 2 medium tomatoes, sliced, on top of the potatoes.

Upside-Down Rice (*Makloubeh*)

In this dish, seasoned rice combines with layers of eggplant and cauliflower and it's all topped with a variety of toasted nuts.

Yield:	Prep time:	Cook time:	Serving size:
8 cups	30 minutes	$1^1/_2$ hours	1 cup
Each serving has:			
247 calories	17g fat	3g saturated fat	9g protein
17g carbohydrate	4g dietary fiber	19mg cholesterol	609mg sodium

1 large eggplant	1 tsp. seven spices
2 tsp. salt	$1/2$ tsp. ground cinnamon
2 cups cauliflower florets	$1/2$ tsp. ground nutmeg
Olive oil spray	$1/2$ tsp. ground cardamom
$1/2$ lb. ground lamb	4 cups water
1 medium yellow onion, finely chopped	$1/3$ cup pine nuts
4 TB. extra-virgin olive oil	$1/3$ cup sliced almonds
$1^1/_2$ cups long-grain rice, rinsed	$1/4$ cup fresh Italian parsley, chopped

1. Preheat the oven to 450°F. Lightly coat a baking sheet with olive oil spray.

2. Cut eggplant into $1/4$-inch slices, sprinkle with $1/2$ teaspoon salt, and let drain in a strainer for 20 minutes. Pat dry.

3. Spread eggplant and cauliflower florets on the prepared baking sheet, lightly coat with olive oil spray, and bake for 20 minutes. Set aside.

4. In a medium skillet over medium heat, brown lamb for 5 minutes, breaking up lumps with a wooden spoon.

5. Add yellow onion and 2 tablespoons extra-virgin olive oil, and cook for 5 minutes.

6. Transfer lamb and onions to a large bowl, and stir in long-grain rice, seven spices, cinnamon, nutmeg, cardamom, and remaining $1^1/_2$ teaspoons salt.

7. In a large, 3-quart pot, add a layer of eggplant, $^1/_2$ of rice mixture, $^1/_2$ of cauliflower, another layer of eggplant, remaining rice mixture, and a final layer of cauliflower. Slowly pour in water, cover, and cook over low heat for 40 minutes. Let rice rest for 15 minutes after cooking.

8. In a small saucepan over low heat, heat remaining 2 tablespoons extra-virgin olive oil. Add pine nuts and almonds, and toast for 3 minutes. Remove from heat.

9. Carefully place a plate over the rice pot, and carefully flip over the pot. Give the pot a few taps and a little jiggle, and slowly lift up the pot.

10. Distribute toasted almonds around the plate, sprinkle Italian parsley over top of rice, and serve warm.

 MEDITERRANEAN MORSEL

If your rice doesn't come out in one piece and falls apart, that's okay. Just decorate the top of the plate with the almonds and the parsley, it will still look, smell, and taste great!

Meat and Rice–Stuffed Grape Leaves

This is a traditional stuffed grape leaves, or *dolma*, recipe. A mixture of meat and rice is rolled in tender grape leaves and cooked in a citrus broth.

Yield:	Prep time:	Cook time:	Serving size:
48 stuffed grape leaves	1 hour, 15 minutes	1^1/$_2$ hours	2 stuffed grape leaves

Each serving has:			
94 calories	5g fat	1g saturated fat	6g protein
7g carbohydrate	0g dietary fiber	11mg cholesterol	1,140mg sodium

2 cups long-grain rice, rinsed	1 (16-oz.) jar grape leaves in brine, drained
1 lb. ground beef	^{1}/$_4$ cup extra-virgin olive oil
2 tsp. salt	6 cups beef broth
1 tsp. ground black pepper	^{1}/$_2$ cup fresh lemon juice
2 TB. minced garlic	

1. In a large bowl, combine long-grain rice, beef, 1 teaspoon salt, black pepper, and garlic.

2. Cover the bottom of a 2-quart pot with a layer of grape leaves. Remove stems from remaining leaves, and place vein side up on your work surface. Spoon 1 tablespoon rice mixture on each leaf, and roll, tucking in edges as you roll. Stack stuffed grape leaves in a circular fashion in the pot.

3. Add extra-virgin olive oil and enough beef broth to cover the top of last stack of grape leaves, and add remaining 1 teaspoon salt. Cover, set over medium-low heat, and simmer for 1^1/$_2$ hours.

4. Remove the pot from heat, and let sit for 30 minutes before serving.

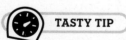 **TASTY TIP**

If the grape leaves are too large, you can cut them in half along the center vein and roll along that horizontal line.

Square Meat Pies (*Sfeeha*)

These little square meat pies contain juicy ground beef with spices nestled in a piece of tender dough.

Yield:	Prep time:	Cook time:	Serving size:
18 meat pies	30 minutes	20 minutes	1 meat pie

Each serving has:			
166 calories	6g fat	2g saturated fat	7g protein
20g carbohydrate	1g dietary fiber	15mg cholesterol	308mg sodium

1 large yellow onion	$^1/_2$ tsp. ground black pepper
2 large tomatoes	1 tsp. seven spices
1 lb. ground beef	1 batch Multipurpose Dough
$1^1/_4$ tsp. salt	(recipe in Chapter 12)

1. Preheat the oven to 425°F.

2. In a food processor fitted with a chopping blade, pulse yellow onion and tomatoes for 30 seconds.

3. Transfer tomato-onion mixture to a large bowl. Add beef, salt, black pepper, and seven spices, and mix well.

4. Form Multipurpose Dough into 18 balls, and roll out to 4-inch circles. Spoon 2 tablespoons meat mixture onto center of each dough circle. Pinch together the two opposite sides of dough up to meat mixture, and pinch the opposite two sides together, forming a square. Place meat pies on a baking sheet, and bake for 20 minutes.

5. Serve warm or at room temperature.

Dumplings in Yogurt Sauce

This is a Mediterranean twist on dumplings. They're cooked in a yogurt sauce and filled with seasoned beef.

Yield:	Prep time:	Cook time:	Serving size:
12 dumplings	20 minutes	30 minutes	2 dumplings

Each serving has:			
412 calories	17g fat	4g saturated fat	32g protein
31g carbohydrate	1g dietary fiber	34mg cholesterol	881mg sodium

1 cup plus 4 TB. all-purpose flour

2^1/$_3$ cups water

5 TB. extra-virgin olive oil

2 tsp. salt

^{1}/$_2$ lb. ground beef

^{1}/$_2$ tsp. ground black pepper

^{1}/$_2$ tsp. seven spices

6 cups plain Greek yogurt

2 TB. cornstarch

2 TB. minced garlic

1 TB. dried mint

1. In a small bowl, knead together 1 cup all-purpose flour, ^{1}/$_3$ cup water, 3 tablespoons extra-virgin olive oil, and ^{1}/$_2$ teaspoon salt. Set aside to rest for 15 minutes.

2. In a small saucepan over medium heat, brown beef for 5 minutes, breaking up chunks with a wooden spoon.

3. Stir in remaining 2 tablespoons extra-virgin olive oil, ^{1}/$_2$ teaspoon salt, black pepper, and seven spices, and cook for 3 more minutes. Set aside.

4. Flour a rolling pin and countertop. Divide dough into 12 pieces, and roll out into 3-inch circles. Place 1 tablespoon meat filling in center of each circle.

5. Using your fingers, dab some water along half of dough circle. Fold dough over filling, forming a half moon, and pinch together dough to seal.

6. In a large pot over medium-low heat, heat Greek yogurt.

7. In a small cup, dissolve cornstarch in remaining 2 cups water. Add to Greek yogurt.

8. Stir in garlic, remaining 1 teaspoon salt, and mint. Bring to a simmer, and cook for about 5 minutes.

9. Reduce heat to low. Drop dumplings into yogurt, and cook for 10 minutes.

10. Serve warm.

MEDITERRANEAN MORSEL

Don't overstir the sauce after you add the dumplings. This could cause the dumplings to break and clump together. Instead, gently move your spoon around the pot two or three times.

Stuffed Squash Casserole

This version of stuffed squash does not include any rice, but instead is zucchini stuffed with seasoned ground beef, toasted pine nuts, and onions and cooked in a zesty tomato sauce.

Yield:	Prep time:	Cook time:	Serving size:
10 stuffed squash	20 minutes	50 minutes	2 stuffed squash

Each serving has:			
447 calories	32g fat	7g saturated fat	24g protein
21g carbohydrate	6g dietary fiber	53mg cholesterol	1,275mg sodium

10 light green summer zucchini	1 tsp. seven spices
4 TB. extra-virgin olive oil	1 (16-oz.) can tomato sauce
1 lb. ground beef	1 cup water
1 large yellow onion, finely chopped	$^1/_2$ tsp. garlic powder
$^1/_2$ cup pine nuts	$^1/_2$ tsp. onion powder
2 tsp. salt	$^1/_2$ tsp. dried oregano
1 tsp. ground black pepper	

1. Preheat the oven to 425°F.

2. Trim off top and core out zucchini. Place zucchini on a baking sheet, and drizzle outsides with 2 tablespoons extra-virgin olive oil. Bake for 15 to 20 minutes, and set aside.

3. In a large skillet over medium heat, brown beef for 5 minutes, breaking up chunks with a wooden spoon.

4. Add yellow onion, pine nuts, remaining 2 tablespoons extra-virgin olive oil, 1 teaspoon salt, $^1/_2$ teaspoon black pepper, and seven spices, and cook for 5 minutes.

5. In a 2-quart pot over medium heat, combine tomato sauce, water, remaining 1 teaspoon salt, remaining $^1/_2$ teaspoon black pepper, garlic powder, onion powder, and oregano, and simmer for 10 minutes.

6. Stuff zucchini with about 3 tablespoons beef mixture each. Place stuffed zucchini in a casserole dish, gently pour tomato sauce over zucchini, and bake for 30 minutes.

7. Serve warm with a side of brown rice.

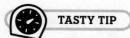 **TASTY TIP**

If you don't like oregano, you can replace it with 2 tablespoons chopped fresh basil.

Beef and Potatoes with Tahini Sauce

This is an easy yet tasty dish to make. Baked ground beef and tender potatoes with a creamy tahini sauce will satisfy your hunger craving.

Yield:	Prep time:	Cook time:	Serving size:
1 (9-inch) casserole	15 minutes	35 minutes	$^1/_6$ of casserole

Each serving has:			
629 calories	4g fat	7g saturated fat	31g protein
40g carbohydrate	6g dietary fiber	48mg cholesterol	1,094mg sodium

$^1/_2$ large yellow onion	2 cups plain Greek yogurt
1 lb. ground beef	$^3/_4$ cup tahini paste
$2^1/_2$ tsp. salt	$1^1/_2$ cups water
$^1/_2$ tsp. ground black pepper	$^1/_4$ cup fresh lemon juice
6 small red potatoes, washed	1 TB. minced garlic
3 TB. extra-virgin olive oil	$^1/_2$ cup pine nuts

1. Preheat the oven to 425°F.

2. In a food processor fitted with a chopping blade, blend yellow onion for 30 seconds.

3. Transfer onion to a large bowl. Add beef, 1 teaspoon salt, black pepper, and mix well.

4. Spread beef mixture evenly in the bottom of a 9-inch casserole dish, and bake for 20 minutes.

5. Cut red potatoes into $^1/_4$-inch-thick pieces, place in a bowl, and toss with 2 tablespoons extra-virgin olive oil and $^1/_2$ teaspoon salt. Spread potatoes on a baking sheet, and bake for 20 minutes.

6. In a large bowl, combine Greek yogurt, tahini paste, water, lemon juice, garlic, and remaining 1 teaspoon salt.

7. Remove beef mixture and potatoes from the oven. Using a spatula, transfer potatoes to the casserole dish. Pour yogurt sauce over top, and bake for 15 more minutes.

8. In a small pan over low heat, heat remaining 1 tablespoon extra-virgin olive oil. Add pine nuts, and toast for 1 or 2 minutes.

9. Remove casserole dish from the oven, spoon pine nuts over top, and serve warm with brown rice.

Stuffed Eggplant Casserole

This dish is a refreshing way to prepare eggplant. Earthy eggplant is filled with browned ground beef and baked in a zesty tomato sauce. Light and full of flavor.

Yield:	Prep time:	Cook time:	Serving size:
10 eggplants	20 minutes	50 minutes	2 eggplants
Each serving has:			
600 calories	33g fat	7g saturated fat	28g protein
61g carbohydrate	33g dietary fiber	53mg cholesterol	1,262mg sodium

10 small Italian eggplants

4 TB. extra-virgin olive oil

1 lb. ground beef

1 large yellow onion, finely chopped

$^1/_2$ cup pine nuts

2 tsp. salt

1 tsp. ground black pepper

1 tsp. seven spices

1 (16-oz.) can tomato sauce

1 cup water

$^1/_2$ tsp. garlic powder

$^1/_2$ tsp. onion powder

$^1/_2$ tsp. dried oregano

1. Preheat the oven to 425°F.

2. Trim off top and peel off some skin from each eggplant. Place eggplants on a baking sheet, drizzle outsides with 2 tablespoons extra-virgin olive oil, bake for 20 minutes. Set aside.

3. In a large skillet over medium heat, brown beef for 5 minutes, breaking up chunks with a wooden spoon.

4. Add yellow onion, pine nuts, remaining 2 tablespoons extra-virgin olive oil, 1 teaspoon salt, $^1/_2$ teaspoon black pepper, and seven spices, and cook for 5 minutes.

5. In a 2-quart pot over medium heat, combine tomato sauce, water, remaining 1 teaspoon salt, remaining $^1/_2$ teaspoon black pepper, garlic powder, onion powder, and oregano, and simmer for 10 minutes.

6. Cut a $1^1/_2$-inch slit in the side of each eggplant, creating a pocket. Stuff pockets with about 3 tablespoons beef mixture.

7. Place stuffed eggplants in a casserole dish, gently pour tomato sauce over eggplants, and bake for 30 minutes.

8. Serve warm with a side of brown rice.

MEDITERRANEAN MORSEL

You can prepare several parts of the **Stuffed Eggplant Casserole** recipe ahead of time so you can pull it all together quickly right before dinner. For example, you can bake the eggplant, cook the filling, and make the tomato sauce in advance and assemble and bake when you're ready.

Lamb Chops

Here, tender lamb chops are flavored with fresh rosemary, a hint of citrus, and garlic and cooked to perfection.

Yield:	Prep time:	Cook time:	Serving size:
6 chops	30 minutes	6 minutes	1 chop

Each serving has:			
232 calories	14g fat	4g saturated fat	23g protein
2g carbohydrate	0g dietary fiber	73mg cholesterol	483mg sodium

6 (³/₄-in.-thick) lamb chops

2 TB. fresh rosemary, finely chopped

3 TB. minced garlic

1 tsp. salt

1 tsp. ground black pepper

3 TB. extra-virgin olive oil

1. In a large bowl, combine lamb chops, rosemary, garlic, salt, black pepper, and extra-virgin olive oil until chops are evenly coated. Let chops marinate at room temperature for at least 25 minutes.

2. Preheat a grill to medium heat.

3. Place chops on the grill, and cook for 3 minutes per side for medium well.

4. Serve warm.

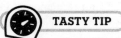

TASTY TIP

If you like your meat well done, leave the lamb chops on the grill for an extra 2 minutes per side.

Roast Leg of Lamb

Juicy, tender roasted lamb seasoned with bright herbs, lemon juice, and aromatic garlic makes for a dinner to remember.

Yield:	Prep time:	Cook time:	Serving size:
60 ounces	10 minutes	2 hours	6 ounces
Each serving has:			
381 calories	20g fat	6g saturated fat	46g protein
2g carbohydrate	0g dietary fiber	145mg cholesterol	578mg sodium

1 (5-lb.) bone-in leg of lamb	2 tsp. salt
10 whole cloves garlic	1 tsp. ground black pepper
2 TB. minced garlic	3 TB. fresh rosemary leaves, finely chopped
$^1/_3$ cup lemon juice	
$^1/_3$ cup extra-virgin olive oil	

1. Preheat the oven to 475°F.

2. Using a sharp paring knife, cut 10 ($^1/_2$-inch) slits into leg of lamb. Stick 1 garlic clove in each slit.

3. In a small bowl, combine garlic, lemon juice, extra-virgin olive oil, salt, black pepper, and rosemary. Rub dressing all over leg of lamb.

4. Place the leg of lamb in a roasting pan, and roast for 30 minutes.

5. Reduce heat to 350°F, and cook for $1^1/_2$ more hours.

6. Remove lamb from the oven and set aside for 20 minutes before cutting and serving.

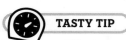 **TASTY TIP**

Whenever you're cooking a large piece of meat, it's always good to cook it low and slow. This helps dissolve the meat's connective tissue, which makes the meat tender.

Lamb Meatballs

Juicy lamb meatballs can be great on their own or in a sandwich with tzatziki sauce.

Yield:	Prep time:	Cook time:	Serving size:
15 meatballs	15 minutes	25 minutes	1 meatball

Each serving has:			
90 calories	7g fat	2g saturated fat	5g protein
2g carbohydrate	0g dietary fiber	20mg cholesterol	173mg sodium

3 TB. extra-virgin olive oil	2 TB. fresh mint, finely chopped
1 large white onion, finely chopped	1 tsp. fresh lemon zest
2 TB. minced garlic	1/2 tsp. ground coriander
1 lb. ground lamb	1/4 tsp. ground cumin
1 tsp. salt	1/4 tsp. ground cinnamon
1/2 tsp. ground black pepper	

1. Preheat the oven to 400°F.

2. In a small skillet over medium heat, heat extra-virgin olive oil. Add white onion and garlic, and cook for 5 minutes.

3. In a medium bowl, combine cooked onions and garlic, lamb, salt, black pepper, mint, lemon zest, coriander, cumin, and cinnamon, breaking up chunks of lamb with a wooden spoon.

4. Form lamb mixture into 15 (2-tablespoons) meatballs. Set meatballs on a baking sheet, and bake for 20 minutes.

5. Remove meatballs from the oven, transfer them to a serving dish, and serve with tzatziki sauce.

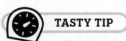 **TASTY TIP**

Feta goes great with lamb meatballs. Add 1/2 cup crumbled feta to your tzatziki sauce to have with the meatballs.

Braised Lamb and Tomatoes

Lamb shanks are wonderful pieces of meat and can be very tender and flavorful. In this recipe, you prepare the lamb shanks by braising them in a zesty tomato sauce.

Yield:	Prep time:	Cook time:	Serving size:
4 lamb shanks	20 minutes	3 hours	1 lamb shank

Each serving has:			
570 calories	31g fat	7g saturated fat	30g protein
44g carbohydrate	6g dietary fiber	80mg cholesterol	2,411mg sodium

$^1/_2$ cup all-purpose flour

4 lamb shanks

2 tsp. salt

$1^1/_2$ tsp. ground black pepper

5 TB. extra-virgin olive oil

1 large yellow onion, finely chopped

5 cloves garlic, finely chopped

1 medium celery stalk, finely chopped

2 large carrots, finely chopped

3 TB. tomato paste

1 (16-oz.) can crushed tomatoes, with juice

5 cups vegetable broth

2 TB. fresh rosemary, finely chopped

2 TB. fresh thyme, finely chopped

1. Place all-purpose flour in a shallow dish.

2. Season lamb shanks with 1 teaspoon salt and $^1/_2$ teaspoon black pepper, and dredge in flour just to coat.

3. In a large, oven-safe pot or a Dutch oven over medium heat, heat 3 tablespoons extra-virgin olive oil. Add lamb shanks, and brown evenly on all sides for about 10 minutes. Remove from the pot.

4. Reduce heat to low, and heat remaining 2 tablespoons extra-virgin olive oil in the pot. Add yellow onion, garlic, celery, and carrots, sauté for 15 minutes.

5. Add tomato paste, and cook for 3 minutes.

6. Add crushed tomatoes with juice, vegetable broth, remaining 1 teaspoon salt, remaining 1 teaspoon black pepper, rosemary, and thyme, and simmer for 5 minutes.

7. Preheat the oven to 400°F.

8. Add lamb shanks to the pot, and pour in more water to cover lamb. Cover the pot, and bake for $2^1/_2$ hours, turning over shanks every 40 minutes, or until meat is very tender and almost falling off the bone.

9. Serve warm with rice.

Lamb and Rice Pockets

Flakey phyllo dough filled with seasoned lamb, rice, and vegetables is a great way to get your protein, carbs, and veggies, all in one convenient pocket.

Yield:	Prep time:	Cook time:	Serving size:
6 pockets	20 minutes	1 hour	1 pocket

Each serving has:			
499 calories	31g fat	14g saturated fat	13g protein
44g carbohydrate	3g dietary fiber	66mg cholesterol	914mg sodium

½ lb. ground lamb	1 tsp. ground black pepper
3 TB. extra-virgin olive oil	1 tsp. seven spices
½ large white onion, chopped	¼ tsp. ground cardamom
4½ cups water	½ tsp. ground cinnamon
1 cup fresh or frozen green peas	2 cups brown basmati rice
2 large carrots, shredded	1 pkg. phyllo dough (12 sheets)
1½ tsp. salt	½ cup butter, melted

1. In a large, 3-quart pot over medium heat, brown lamb for 5 minutes, breaking up chunks with a wooden spoon.

2. Add extra-virgin olive oil and white onion, and cook for 5 minutes.

3. Add water, green peas, carrots, salt, black pepper, seven spices, cardamom, and cinnamon, and bring to a simmer.

4. Add brown basmati rice, cover, reduce heat to low, and cook for 40 minutes.

5. Preheat the oven to 400°F.

6. Place first sheet of phyllo on your work surface, brush with melted butter, lay second sheet of phyllo on top, and brush with melted butter. Cut phyllo into 10×10-inch squares.

7. Spoon 1 cup rice mixture into center of phyllo square, and fold each side over to form a square. Place pocket on a baking sheet, and brush top with butter. Bake for 15 to 20 minutes or until pockets are golden brown.

8. Serve warm with a side of Greek yogurt.

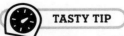 **TASTY TIP**

If you don't like carrots or peas, you can substitute your choice of vegetable instead. Try broccoli or asparagus, for example. Just be sure to chop whatever you decide to use small.

Chicken Entrées

Chicken is one of the most popular proteins consumed in the Mediterranean region, in part because it's relatively inexpensive and very versatile. Chicken can be cooked whole, with skin or without, and with bones or boneless. In this chapter, you learn some preparation techniques that will enable you to explore new flavor combinations.

One fear many people have when cooking chicken, is undercooking it or cooking it so much it becomes dry. Therefore, using a cooking thermometer is a good idea. In general, chicken should be cooked to an internal temperature of between 165°F and 175°F, depending on the cut of chicken, whether it's the breast or thighs. Also keep in mind what's called *carryover heat,* or when the chicken continues to cook after you remove it from the heat source. Due to carryover heat, the temperature of the chicken will continue to rise 5 to 10 degrees, so be sure to remove your chicken immediately from heat when it hits that 165°F degree temperature. As soon as you get a hang of how long to cook your chicken, your dishes will never be dry again.

In This Chapter

- Pleasing poultry dishes
- Flavorful chicken meals
- No more dry, bland chicken

Chicken Shawarma

This recipe is the opposite of flavorless chicken. In this dish, the chicken is marinated in an array of pungent spices and cooked to perfection.

Yield:	Prep time:	Cook time:	Serving size:
1 pound	30 minutes	15 minutes	$^1/_4$ pound

Each serving has:			
271 calories	16g fat	2g saturated fat	28g protein
4g carbohydrate	1g dietary fiber	65mg cholesterol	515mg sodium

1 lb. boneless, skinless chicken breast	$^1/_2$ tsp. cayenne
$^1/_4$ cup fresh lemon juice	$^1/_2$ tsp. paprika
$^1/_4$ cup Greek yogurt	1 tsp. dried parsley
2 TB. minced garlic	4 TB. extra-virgin olive oil
$^1/_2$ tsp. seven spices	$^3/_4$ tsp. salt
$^1/_4$ tsp. ground cardamom	$^1/_2$ tsp. ground black pepper
$^1/_4$ tsp. ground cinnamon	

1. Using a sharp knife, cut chicken into thin, $^1/_4$-inch strips. Place strips in a large bowl.

2. Add lemon juice, Greek yogurt, garlic, seven spices, cardamom, cinnamon, cayenne, paprika, parsley, extra-virgin olive oil, salt, and black pepper.

3. Marinate chicken in the refrigerator for at least 20 minutes and up to 24 hours.

4. In a large skillet over medium heat, cook chicken and marinade for 20 minutes or until chicken is lightly browned and marinade has evaporated.

5. Serve warm with pita bread and garlic sauce.

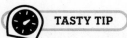 **TASTY TIP**

You can save time with this recipe by prepping and marinating it the day before you plan to have it for lunch or dinner.

Spiced Chicken and Rice

This dish is full of eastern spices, tender chicken, fluffy rice, and the crunch of toasted nuts.

Yield:	Prep time:	Cook time:	Serving size:
8 cups	30 minutes	$1^1/_2$ hours	1 cup

Each serving has:			
357 calories	23g fat	3g saturated fat	12g protein
28g carbohydrate	4g dietary fiber	20mg cholesterols	986mg sodium

2 whole chicken thighs, including drumstick, skin, and bones

$^1/_2$ large yellow onion, quartered

1 (3-in.) cinnamon stick

2 bay leaves

2 tsp. salt

8 cups water

3 TB. plus 2 tsp. extra-virgin olive oil

1 medium yellow onion, finely chopped

1 large ripe tomato, finely chopped

2 cups long-grain rice, rinsed

$^1/_2$ tsp. ground cardamom

$^1/_2$ tsp. ground cloves

$^1/_2$ tsp. seven spices

$^1/_2$ tsp. ground nutmeg

$^1/_2$ tsp. ground cinnamon

$^1/_2$ tsp. ground black pepper

4 cups chicken broth

$^1/_2$ cup sliced almonds

$^1/_2$ cup pistachios

$^1/_2$ cup pine nuts

$^1/_2$ cup white or golden raisins

1. In a large pot over medium heat, bring chicken, yellow quartered onion, cinnamon stick, bay leaves, 1 teaspoon salt, and water to a boil. Cook, skimming off any foam, for 40 minutes. Set aside to cool. Remove chicken from broth, and pull apart chicken, discarding skin and bones.

2. In another large pot over medium heat, heat 3 tablespoons extra-virgin olive oil. Add chopped yellow onion and tomato, and cook, stirring intermittently, for 7 minutes.

3. Add long-grain rice, cardamom, cloves, seven spices, nutmeg, cinnamon, and black pepper to onion-tomato mixture, and cook, stirring intermittently, for 3 minutes.

4. Add chicken broth from the pot to rice mixture, and stir. Reduce heat to low, cover, and cook for 40 minutes.

5. Remove from heat, fluff rice with a fork, cover, and set aside for 10 minutes.

6. In a small saucepan over low heat, heat remaining 2 teaspoons extra-virgin olive oil. Add almonds, pistachios, pine nuts, and white raisins, and toast for 3 minutes. Set aside.

7. To serve, spoon rice onto a serving dish. Top rice with chicken and toasted nuts, and serve warm.

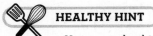 **HEALTHY HINT**

You can make this dish a bit healthier by using brown basmati rice instead of white long-grain rice.

Chicken Roulade

This is a visually beautiful and flavorful chicken roll filled with sautéed vegetables and a smooth ricotta cheese.

Yield:	Prep time:	Cook time:	Serving size:
12 slices	20 minutes	50 minutes	1 slice

Each serving has:			
238 calories	13g fat	5g saturated fat	25g protein
6g carbohydrate	1g dietary fiber	96mg cholesterol	648mg sodium

4 TB. extra-virgin olive oil

6 cups fresh spinach, chopped

1 large red bell pepper, roasted, ribs and seeds removed, and chopped

2 lb. ground chicken

2 tsp. salt

1 tsp. ground black pepper

1 tsp. garlic powder

1 tsp. paprika

$1/2$ tsp. onion powder

$1/2$ cup plain breadcrumbs

1 lb. ricotta cheese

1 cup shredded Parmesan cheese

$1/2$ cup fresh Italian parsley, chopped

1. Preheat the oven to 425°F. Evenly spray a 9×5-inch bread loaf pan with olive oil spray.

2. In a large skillet over medium heat, heat 2 tablespoons extra-virgin olive oil. Add spinach, and cook for 3 minutes.

3. Add roasted red bell pepper, and cook for 2 minutes. Set aside.

4. In a large bowl, combine chicken, salt, black pepper, garlic powder, paprika, onion powder, and breadcrumbs.

5. Lay out a long, 30×10-inch piece of parchment or waxed paper on your counter, and spray with olive oil spray.

6. Spread chicken mixture onto the paper and shape into a rectangle slightly smaller than the size of the paper.

7. Evenly distribute spinach and red bell pepper over chicken, followed by ricotta cheese, Parmesan cheese, and Italian parsley.

8. Gently pull one end of the paper up and forward, causing end of chicken to fold over, and continue to pull the paper forward, allowing chicken to roll up into a loaf.

9. Place chicken loaf in the prepared bread loaf pan, and drizzle with remaining 2 tablespoons extra-virgin olive oil. Cover the pan with aluminum foil, and bake for 35 minutes.

10. Remove the foil, and cook for 5 more minutes.

11. Let loaf rest for 15 minutes. Slice loaf, revealing the pinwheel appearance of chicken, cheese, and vegetables, and serve warm.

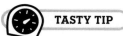 **TASTY TIP**

If you like a more pungent cheese, add some goat cheese to the filling along with some olives, finely chopped and pitted.

Roasted Chicken

This beautiful roasted chicken with a crispy skin is flavored with spices and herbs and is accompanied by sweet roasted carrots.

Yield:	Prep time:	Cook time:	Serving size:
1 whole chicken	10 minutes	1 hour, 15 minutes	$^1/_4$ chicken

Each serving has:			
611 calories	18g fat	5g saturated fat	59g protein
50g carbohydrate	6g dietary fiber	160mg cholesterol	795mg sodium

1 (5-lb.) whole chicken	$^1/_2$ large lemon, cut in $^1/_2$
1 TB. extra-virgin olive oil	$^1/_2$ large yellow onion, cut in $^1/_2$
2 TB. minced garlic	2 sprigs fresh rosemary
1 tsp. salt	2 sprigs fresh thyme
1 tsp. paprika	2 sprigs fresh sage
1 tsp. black pepper	2 large carrots, cut into 1-in. pieces
1 tsp. ground coriander	6 small red potatoes, washed and cut in $^1/_2$
1 tsp. seven spices	4 cloves garlic
$^1/_2$ tsp. ground cinnamon	

1. Preheat the oven to 450°F. Wash chicken and pat dry with paper towels. Place chicken in a roasting pan, and drizzle and then rub chicken with extra-virgin olive oil.

2. In a small bowl, combine garlic, salt, paprika, black pepper, coriander, seven spices, and cinnamon. Sprinkle and then rub entire chicken with spice mixture to coat.

3. Place $^1/_4$ lemon, $^1/_4$ yellow onion, 1 sprig rosemary, 1 sprig thyme, and 1 sprig sage in chicken cavity.

4. Place remaining rosemary, thyme, sage, lemon, and onion around chicken in the roasting pan. Add carrots, red potatoes, and garlic cloves to the roasting pan.

5. Roast for 15 minutes. Reduce temperature to 375°F, and roast for 1 more hour, basting chicken every 20 minutes.

6. Let chicken rest for 15 minutes before serving.

Mediterranean Meatloaf

This recipe puts a Mediterranean twist on traditional meatloaf, integrating fresh herbs and spices with ground chicken, which makes it a bit more healthy as well.

Yield:	Prep time:	Cook time:	Serving size:
1 (9×5-inch) loaf	15 minutes	45 minutes	$^1/_8$ loaf

Each serving has:			
302 calories	14g fat	4g saturated fat	30g protein
17g carbohydrate	1g dietary fiber	148mg cholesterol	975mg sodium

2 lb. ground chicken	2 TB. fresh basil, chopped
$^1/_3$ cup plain breadcrumbs	2 TB. fresh Italian parsley, chopped
$1^1/_2$ tsp. salt	1 large egg
1 tsp. garlic powder	1 large carrot, shredded
1 tsp. ground black pepper	1 cup fresh or frozen green peas
1 tsp. paprika	$^1/_2$ cup sun-dried tomatoes, chopped
$^1/_2$ tsp. dried oregano	1 cup ketchup
$^1/_2$ tsp. dried thyme	

1. Preheat the oven to 400°F. Lightly coat all sides of a 9×5-inch loaf pan with olive oil spray.

2. In a large bowl, combine chicken, breadcrumbs, salt, garlic powder, black pepper, paprika, oregano, thyme, basil, Italian parsley, egg, carrot, green peas, and sun-dried tomatoes.

3. Transfer chicken mixture to the prepared pan, and even out top. Cover the pan with a piece of aluminum foil, and bake for 40 minutes.

4. After 40 minutes have passed, pour ketchup over top of loaf and spread out evenly. Bake for 5 more minutes.

5. Remove meatloaf from the oven, and let rest for 10 minutes before slicing and serving warm.

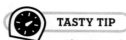 **TASTY TIP**

If you're a fan of turkey, this is a great recipe to replace the ground chicken with ground turkey.

Chicken Kefta Kabob

These kabobs are a great way to make flavorful ground chicken with little fat but a lot of flavor.

Yield:	Prep time:	Cook time:	Serving size:
8 kabobs	10 minutes	7 minutes	1 kabob
Each serving has:			
113 calories	6g fat	2g saturated fat	13g protein
1g carbohydrate	0g dietary fiber	61mg cholesterol	336mg sodium

$^1/_2$ medium yellow onion	$^1/_2$ tsp. paprika
$^1/_2$ cup fresh Italian parsley	$^1/_4$ tsp. ground cumin
1 lb. ground chicken	$^1/_4$ tsp. ground coriander
1 tsp. salt	$^1/_4$ tsp. ground cinnamon
$^1/_2$ tsp. ground black pepper	

1. Preheat the grill to medium heat.

2. In a food processor fitted with a chopping blade, blend yellow onion and Italian parsley for 30 seconds.

3. Transfer onion-parsley mixture to a large bowl. Add chicken, salt, black pepper, paprika, cumin, coriander, cinnamon, and mix well.

4. Form chicken mixture into 8 (3-inch) kabobs using 3 tablespoons chicken mixture each.

5. Add kabobs to the grill, and cook for 3 minutes without touching to prevent kabobs from breaking. Rotate kabobs, and grill for 3 more minutes. Rotate one more time, and cook for 2 minutes. Serve warm with a side of hummus.

MEDITERRANEAN MORSEL

When forming the chicken mixture into finger-size kabobs, add a few drops of water to your hands to prevent the chicken from sticking. This also makes it easier to form the chicken into kabobs.

Chicken Skewers (*Shish Tawook*)

These chicken skewers look good and taste even better. The paprika gives this dish a beautiful orange color and smoky flavor with a hint of citrus.

Yield:	Prep time:	Cook time:	Serving size:
5 skewers	30 minutes	8 minutes	1 skewer

Each serving has:			
244 calories	11g fat	2g saturated fat	33g protein
4g carbohydrate	1g dietary fiber	77mg cholesterol	561mg sodium

1¹/₂ lb. boneless, skinless chicken breasts	2 TB. tomato paste
2 TB. minced garlic	1 TB. paprika
3 TB. fresh lemon juice	¹/₂ tsp. cayenne
3 TB. extra-virgin olive oil	1 tsp. salt
2 TB. Greek yogurt	¹/₂ tsp. ground black pepper

1. Preheat a grill to medium heat.

2. Cut chicken breast into 1-inch cubes and place in a large bowl.

3. Add garlic, lemon juice, extra-virgin olive oil, Greek yogurt, tomato paste, paprika, cayenne, salt, and black pepper, and mix to combine.

4. Skewer chicken, dividing equally among 5 skewers. Place chicken on the grill, and cook for 8 minutes, turning over every 2 minutes to grill all sides.

5. Serve warm with hummus and pita bread.

TASTY TIP

Depending on if you like your food to be spicy or not, you can reduce or increase the cayenne in this recipe to suit your taste.

Chicken and Potatoes

In this warm and filling dish, garlic and lemon seasoned chicken and potatoes are baked to perfection.

Yield:	Prep time:	Cook time:	Serving size:
6 drumsticks and 6 potatoes	15 minutes	50 minutes	1 drumstick and 1 potato

Each serving has:			
331 calories	15g fat	3g saturated fat	18g protein
31g carbohydrate	3g dietary fiber	47mg cholesterol	646mg sodium

6 chicken drumsticks, skin on

6 small red potatoes, washed and cut into quarters

4 TB. minced garlic

$^1/_2$ cup lemon juice

$^1/_4$ cup extra-virgin olive oil

$1^1/_2$ tsp. salt

1 tsp. ground black pepper

1 tsp. paprika

$^1/_2$ tsp. cayenne

1. Preheat the oven to 450°F.

2. In a large roasting pan, add chicken and red potatoes.

3. In a small bowl, combine garlic, lemon juice, extra-virgin olive oil, salt, black pepper, paprika, and cayenne. Pour dressing over chicken and potatoes, and toss to combine.

4. Cover the pan with aluminum foil, and bake for 30 minutes.

5. Remove the foil, and roast for 15 more minutes.

6. Serve warm.

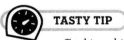 **TASTY TIP**

Cooking chicken with the bone in keeps the chicken moist and gives it more flavor.

Braised Chicken

You are guaranteed a juicy and flavorful piece of chicken and sauce with this tasty chicken recipe.

Yield:	Prep time:	Cook time:	Serving size:
6 drumsticks	10 minutes	52 minutes	1 drumstick

Each serving has:			
176 calories	10g fat	2g saturated fat	14g protein
9g carbohydrate	1g dietary fiber	41mg cholesterol	703mg sodium

6 chicken drumsticks, skin on	1 tsp. ground black pepper
3 TB. extra-virgin olive oil	2 cups water
2 cups crimini mushrooms, cleaned	2 TB. tomato paste
1 large yellow onion, chopped	$^1/_3$ cup tomato sauce
12 cloves garlic	1 TB. brown sugar, packed
$1^1/_2$ tsp. salt	$^1/_2$ tsp. cayenne

1. In a large, 3-quart pot over medium heat, brown chicken drumsticks for 10 minutes, rotating every 3 minutes. Remove chicken from the pot, and set aside.

2. In the pot, combine extra-virgin olive oil, crimini mushrooms, yellow onion, garlic, and salt. Cook for 7 minutes.

3. Add black pepper, water, tomato paste, tomato sauce, brown sugar, and cayenne, and simmer for 5 minutes.

4. Return chicken to the pot, reduce heat to low, cover, and simmer for 30 minutes.

5. Serve each drumstick with sauce and some vegetables.

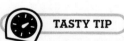 **TASTY TIP**

This recipe goes great with brown rice, plain pasta, or even one of the pilaf recipes in this book.

Grilled Chicken on the Bone

Grilling chicken on the bone ensures you get juicy, tender chicken with a nice, smoky grill flavor.

Yield:	Prep time:	Cook time:	Serving size:
4 drumsticks and 4 thighs	1 hour	40 minutes	1 drumstick and 1 thigh

Each serving has:			
451 calories	35g fat	6g saturated fat	27g protein
7g carbohydrate	1g dietary fiber	90mg cholesterol	1,253mg sodium

4 TB. minced garlic	1 tsp. ground black pepper
$1/2$ cup fresh lemon juice	1 tsp. cayenne
$1/2$ cup extra-virgin olive oil	1 tsp. paprika
1 TB. dried oregano	4 chicken drumsticks
2 tsp. salt	4 chicken thighs

1. In a small bowl, whisk together garlic, lemon juice, extra-virgin olive oil, oregano, salt, black pepper, cayenne, and paprika.

2. Place chicken drumsticks and chicken thighs in a large bowl, pour $1/2$ of dressing over chicken, mix to coat evenly, and set in the refrigerator to marinate for 1 hour.

3. Preheat the grill to medium-high heat.

4. Place chicken evenly on the grill, and cook for 5 minutes per side.

5. Reduce heat to medium-low, cover the grill, and cook chicken for 15 minutes per side or until juices run clear and internal temperature of chicken reads 175°F.

6. Remove chicken from the grill, and let rest for 5 minutes before serving warm.

Seafood Suppers

If you like seafood as the star ingredient in your main dish, this is the chapter for you. Whether it's shrimp, cod, tilapia, haddock, or salmon, seafood is good for you, thanks to its omega-3 fatty acid content.

Fish is a popular protein in Mediterranean countries and an integral part of the Mediterranean diet. With the close proximity of the Mediterranean Sea, seafood is fresh and convenient—and an important industry for the local economy.

Many people are hesitant when cooking fish because they don't know how or they're afraid of the smell. But it's actually pretty simple. The only reason that fish should smell is if it's not fresh or if you overcook it, destroying the fatty acids it contains. Most fish cooks in a matter of minutes on the stovetop, so watch that you don't cook it too long.

Be sure to find a good seafood supplier and follow the recipe cooking directions, and you should be on your way to reaping the benefits of seafood.

In This Chapter

- Delightful dishes from the sea
- Simple, sensational seafood
- Spiced and sauced dishes

Fish and Rice (*Sayadieh*)

This dish has an array of spices and some sweetness from the onions. The rice is fluffy and well seasoned with perfectly cooked pieces of fish.

Yield:	Prep time:	Cook time:	Serving size:
8 cups	30 minutes	$1^1/_2$ hours	1 cup

Each serving has:			
293 calories	18g fat	2g saturated fat	17g protein
17g carbohydrate	2g dietary fiber	44mg cholesterol	621mg sodium

1 lb. whitefish fillets (cod, tilapia, or haddock)

2 tsp. salt

2 tsp. ground black pepper

$^1/_4$ cup plus 2 TB. extra-virgin olive oil

2 large yellow onions, sliced

5 cups water

1 tsp. turmeric

1 tsp. ground coriander

$^1/_2$ tsp. ground cumin

$^1/_4$ tsp. ground cinnamon

2 cups basmati rice

$^1/_2$ cup sliced almonds

1. Season both sides of whitefish with 1 teaspoon salt and 1 teaspoon black pepper.

2. In a skillet over medium heat, heat $^1/_4$ cup extra-virgin olive oil. Add fish, and cook for 3 minutes per side. Remove fish from the pan.

3. Add yellow onions to the skillet, reduce heat to medium-low, and cook for 15 minutes or until golden brown and caramelized.

4. In a 3-quart pot over medium heat, add $^1/_2$ of cooked onions, water, turmeric, coriander, cumin, cinnamon, remaining 1 teaspoon salt, and remaining 1 teaspoon black pepper. Simmer for 20 minutes.

5. Add basmati rice, cover, and cook for 30 minutes.

6. Cut fish into $^1/_2$-inch pieces, fluff rice, and gently fold fish into rice. Cover and cook for 10 more minutes.

7. Remove from heat, and let sit for 10 minutes before serving.

8. Meanwhile, in a small saucepan over low heat, heat remaining 2 tablespoons extra-virgin olive oil. Add almonds, and toast for 3 minutes.

9. Spoon fish and rice onto a serving plate, top with remaining onions and toasted almonds, and serve.

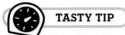 **TASTY TIP**

In the Fish and Rice recipe, you can use brown basmati rice instead of white basmati rice. The brown rice also adds a nice, earthy flavor to the dish.

Spiced Fish

This fish really has a kick! Baked flakey red snapper is seasoned with a spicy vegetable sauce in this eye-opening fish dish.

Yield:	Prep time:	Cook time:	Serving size:
1 (6-pound) fish	15 minutes	1 hour	$^1/_4$ fish

Each serving has:			
450 calories	24g fat	4g saturated fat	47g protein
11g carbohydrate	2g dietary fiber	80mg cholesterol	984mg sodium

1 large ripe tomato	2 TB. tomato paste
1 large yellow onion	3 TB. fresh lemon juice
1 jalapeño, some seeds removed	$^1/_4$ cup plus 2 TB. extra-virgin olive oil
4 cloves garlic	
$^1/_2$ cup plus 2 TB. fresh cilantro	1 (6-lb.) whole red snapper, scales and guts removed
1 tsp. ground cumin	6 lemon slices
1 tsp. ground coriander	$^1/_2$ large lemon
$1^1/_2$ tsp. salt	
1 tsp. ground black pepper	

1. Preheat the oven to 375°F.

2. In a food processor fitted with a chopping blade, pulse tomato, yellow onion, jalapeño, garlic, $^1/_2$ cup cilantro, cumin, coriander, 1 teaspoon salt, $^1/_2$ teaspoon black pepper, tomato paste, lemon juice, and $^1/_4$ cup extra-virgin olive oil 15 times.

3. Place 3 slices of lemon in a roasting pan, and set red snapper on top. Gently squeeze and scrub top of fish with $^1/_2$ lemon, and pat dry with a paper towel.

4. Drizzle remaining 2 tablespoons extra-virgin olive oil over fish, and season with remaining $^1/_2$ teaspoon salt and remaining $^1/_2$ teaspoon black pepper.

5. Spoon vegetable filling inside fish. (It's okay if some of it leaks out.) Top fish with remaining 3 lemon slices, and cover the pan with aluminum foil.

6. Bake for 45 minutes. Remove the foil, and bake for 10 more minutes.

7. Let fish rest for 10 minutes, sprinkle with remaining 2 tablespoons cilantro, and serve on a bed of rice.

Pan-Seared Cod with Cherry Tomatoes

Cod is a nice, flakey whitefish. In this recipe, it's seared to perfection and topped with flavorful bursts of cherry tomatoes and cooked spinach.

Yield:	Prep time:	Cook time:	Serving size:
2 fillets	15 minutes	17 minutes	1 fillet

Each serving has:			
516 calories	36g fat	8g saturated fat	41g protein
8g carbohydrate	2g dietary fiber	111mg cholesterol	2,291mg sodium

2 (6-oz.) cod fillets	1 TB. garlic, minced
1¹/₂ tsp. salt	2 cups fresh spinach
1 tsp. ground black pepper	3 TB. capers, drained
4 TB. extra-virgin olive oil	2 TB. fresh Italian parsley, finely chopped
1 TB. unsalted butter	
1 cup cherry tomatoes	2 TB. fresh lemon juice

1. Season both sides of cod fillets with 1 teaspoon salt and ¹/₂ teaspoon black pepper.

2. In a large, nonstick skillet over medium heat, heat 2 tablespoons extra-virgin olive oil and unsalted butter. When butter is melted, add cod, and cook for 5 minutes per side. Remove to a serving plate.

3. Add remaining 2 tablespoons extra-virgin olive oil, cherry tomatoes, and garlic. Cook for 2 minutes.

4. Add spinach, and cook for 3 minutes.

5. Add remaining ¹/₂ teaspoon salt, remaining ¹/₂ teaspoon black pepper, capers, Italian parsley, and lemon juice, and cook for 2 minutes.

6. Spoon spinach mixture over cod fillets, and serve warm.

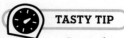 **TASTY TIP**

Capers have a nice, briny flavor, but if you don't have or like capers, you can replace them with green olives. Either ingredient adds a bit of a pungent flavor to the gentle fish flavor.

Salmon with Pesto

Here, sizzling seared salmon is topped with a light and flavorful herb pesto.

Yield:	Prep time:	Cook time:	Serving size:
2 fillets	20 minutes	10 minutes	1 fillet

Each serving has:			
403 calories	26g fat	5g saturated fat	24g protein
20g carbohydrate	5g dietary fiber	70mg cholesterol	1,181mg sodium

2 cups fresh basil	3 TB. toasted pine nuts
2 cloves garlic	$^1/_4$ cup plus 2 TB. extra-virgin olive oil
4 TB. fresh lemon juice	2 (6-oz.) salmon fillets
1 tsp. salt	$^1/_2$ medium lemon
1 tsp. ground black pepper	
3 TB. grated Parmesan cheese	

1. In a food processor fitted with a chopping blade, pulse basil, garlic, 2 tablespoons lemon juice, $^1/_2$ teaspoon salt, and $^1/_2$ teaspoon black pepper 15 times.

2. Add Parmesan cheese, pine nuts, and $^1/_4$ cup extra-virgin olive oil, and pulse 15 more times. Set aside.

3. Set salmon fillets on a plate. Drizzle both sides with remaining 2 tablespoons lemon juice, and season with remaining $^1/_2$ teaspoon salt and remaining $^1/_2$ teaspoon black pepper.

4. In a large, nonstick skillet over medium heat, heat remaining 2 tablespoons extra-virgin olive oil. Add salmon, and cook for 5 minutes per side.

5. Place salmon on a serving plate, spoon 2 tablespoons pesto over each piece, and serve warm.

Baked Salmon

This is a quick and easy way to make flavorful salmon without all the fuss—or the fat and calories you'd get from the butter and oil you'd need to fry the fish.

Yield:	Prep time:	Cook time:	Serving size:
4 fillets	10 minutes	13 minutes	1 fillet

Each serving has:			
394 calories	25g fat	5g saturated fat	38g protein
2g carbohydrate	0g dietary fiber	107mg cholesterol	686mg sodium

1 tsp. salt	¹/₂ tsp. dried thyme
1 tsp. ground black pepper	4 (6-oz.) salmon fillets
1 tsp. garlic powder	4 tsp. fresh lemon juice
1 tsp. dried oregano	4 tsp. extra-virgin olive oil
1 tsp. paprika	

1. Preheat the oven to 400°F. Line a baking sheet with aluminum foil.

2. In a small bowl, combine salt, black pepper, garlic powder, oregano, paprika, and thyme.

3. Place salmon fillets on the prepared baking sheet. Drizzle each fillet with 1 teaspoon lemon juice and 1 teaspoon extra-virgin olive oil. Generously season both sides of salmon with seasoning mixture.

4. Bake for 10 minutes.

5. Turn on the broiler, move the baking sheet under the broiler, and cook for 3 minutes.

6. Serve with balsamic vinegar and brown rice.

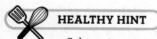 **HEALTHY HINT**

Salmon is easy to prepare and a great source of protein and omega-3 fatty acids. Eating salmon twice a week can help control cholesterol and improve brain function.

Tilapia with a Light Olive Sauce

This pan-seared tilapia is paired with a light sauce that's flavored with pungent black olives and crisp, fresh asparagus.

Yield:	Prep time:	Cook time:	Serving size:
2 fillets	20 minutes	20 minutes	1 fillet

Each serving has:			
631 calories	46g fat	8g saturated fat	45g protein
15g carbohydrate	2g dietary fiber	111mg cholesterol	1,615mg sodium

4 TB. extra-virgin olive oil

1 whole leek, chopped

1 TB. garlic, minced

1 tsp. salt

1 tsp. ground black pepper

1 cup kalamata olives, pitted and sliced

4 stalks asparagus, chopped into 1-in. pieces

1 TB. fresh tarragon, chopped

1 tsp. lemon zest

3 TB. fresh lemon juice

1 TB. unsalted butter

2 (6-oz.) tilapia fillets

1. In a large skillet over medium heat, heat 2 tablespoons extra-virgin olive oil. Add leek, garlic, $^1/_2$ teaspoon salt, and $^1/_2$ teaspoon black pepper, and cook for 3 minutes.

2. Add kalamata olives, asparagus, tarragon, and lemon zest, and cook for 3 minutes.

3. Stir in lemon juice and unsalted butter, and cook for 2 minutes. Set aside.

4. Season both sides of the tilapia with remaining $^1/_2$ teaspoon salt and remaining $^1/_2$ teaspoon black pepper.

5. In a medium nonstick skillet over medium heat, heat remaining 2 tablespoons extra-virgin olive oil. Add tilapia, and cook for 3 minutes per side.

6. Place tilapia on a serving dish, spoon olive-vegetable mixture on top, and serve warm.

Vegetarian Entrées

Plants are an essential part of the Mediterranean diet pyramid. Vegetables are easy to find in most areas, and they're much more inexpensive than meat. The best part is, there are so many vegetables to choose from. Try visiting your local farmers' market and explore the fresh, in-season vegetables available at their peak of freshness and flavor.

In this chapter, you'll see that combining a vegetable with a grain can make for a very interesting meal that not only tastes good but also fills you up and makes you forget you didn't eat any meat.

Another great thing about vegetables is that they're a great base upon which to try different spices and herbs. If you want to try a new spice, try sautéing some potatoes with onion in some extra-virgin olive oil, and sample your new spice with it. This gives you a good gauge of what you can use the spice for and opens your mind to many possibilities.

In This Chapter

- Versatile vegetarian dishes
- Veggie and grain main dishes
- Vegetarian kibbeh and rolls

Vegetarian Quinoa Pilaf

Quinoa is an amazing superfood. This nutty-tasting seed is full of protein and fiber. This pilaf dish combines the earthy flavor of quinoa with sweet tomatoes and pungent olives.

Yield:	Prep time:	Cook time:	Serving size:
8 cups	20 minutes	35 minutes	1 cup

Each serving has:			
129 calories	6g fat	1g saturated fat	3g protein
16g carbohydrate	3g dietary fiber	0mg cholesterol	661mg sodium

3 TB. extra-virgin olive oil

2 portobello mushrooms, sliced

1 medium red onion, finely chopped

1 TB. minced garlic

1 (16-oz.) can diced tomatoes, with juice

2 cups water

2 tsp. salt

1 TB. dried oregano

1 TB. turmeric

1 tsp. paprika

1 tsp. ground black pepper

2 cups red or yellow quinoa

1/2 cup fresh parsley, chopped

1. In a large, 3-quart pot over medium heat, heat extra-virgin olive oil. Add portobello mushrooms, and cook for 5 minutes.

2. Add red onion and garlic, stir, and cook for 5 minutes.

3. Add tomatoes with juice, water, salt, oregano, turmeric, paprika, and black pepper. Stir, and simmer for 5 minutes.

4. Add red quinoa to the pot, and stir. Cover, reduce heat to low, and cook for 20 minutes.

5. Remove from heat, fluff with a fork, cover, and let sit for 10 minutes.

6. Spoon quinoa onto a plate, sprinkle with parsley, and serve warm.

Vegetarian Bowtie Veggie Pasta

This is a nice and light pasta dish with peppery arugula and tangy sun-dried tomatoes.

Yield:	Prep time:	Cook time:	Serving size:
12 cups	20 minutes	20 minutes	1 cup
Each serving has:			
102 calories	5g fat	2g saturated fat	3g protein
12g carbohydrate	1g dietary fiber	18mg cholesterol	442mg sodium

2 tsp. salt

1 lb. bowtie pasta

2 TB. extra-virgin olive oil

2 cups crimini mushrooms, cleaned and sliced

2 TB. minced garlic

1 cup broccoli florets

$^{1}/_{2}$ cup sun-dried tomatoes

2 TB. unsalted butter

2 cups fresh arugula

1 tsp. black pepper

1 tsp. crushed red pepper flakes

1. Bring a large pot of water to a boil over high heat. Add 1 teaspoon salt and bowtie pasta, stir, and cook for 8 minutes.

2. In a large skillet over medium heat, heat extra-virgin olive oil. Add crimini mushrooms, and cook for 4 minutes.

3. Add garlic, broccoli, and sun-dried tomatoes, and cook for 3 minutes.

4. Add remaining 1 teaspoon salt, unsalted butter, arugula, black pepper, and crushed red pepper flakes. Toss, and cook for 2 minutes.

5. Using a slotted spoon, transfer pasta to the skillet, toss pasta with vegetables, and serve warm.

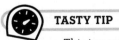 **TASTY TIP**

This is a great recipe to use to incorporate more vegetables into your kids' meals. Try adding spinach or asparagus.

Vegetarian Couscous-Stuffed Tomatoes

I love this dish because it looks so pretty and smells absolutely amazing. Nutty bulgur wheat, seasoned with herbs, and crunchy pine nuts.

Yield:	Prep time:	Cook time:	Serving size:
4 tomatoes	30 minutes	40 minutes	1 tomato

Each serving has:			
321 calories	26g fat	3g saturated fat	6g protein
22g carbohydrate	6g dietary fiber	0mg cholesterol	1,178mg sodium

1 cup bulgur wheat, grind #2, rinsed	2 TB. fresh parsley, chopped
2 cups hot water	1 tsp. seven spices
4 TB. extra-virgin olive oil	$1/2$ tsp. ground nutmeg
1 medium yellow onion, finely chopped	2 tsp. salt
$1/2$ cup pine nuts	2 tsp. ground black pepper
2 TB. fresh dill, chopped	$1/2$ cup water

1. In a medium bowl, place bulgur wheat. Pour hot water over bulgur, and let sit for 20 minutes.

2. Cut off top quarter of tomatoes, and hollow out insides, removing ribs and seeds. Chop tomato tops.

3. In a small skillet over medium heat, heat 2 tablespoons extra-virgin olive oil. Add yellow onion and chopped tomatoes, and cook for 5 minutes.

4. Add pine nuts, and cook for 3 minutes.

5. Transfer onion mixture to the bowl with bulgur. Add dill, parsley, seven spices, nutmeg, 1 teaspoon salt, and 1 teaspoon black pepper, and mix well.

6. Preheat the oven to 400°F.

7. Season inside of tomatoes with remaining 1 teaspoon salt and 1 teaspoon black pepper. Spoon bulgur mixture into tomatoes, filling them to the top.

8. Place tomatoes in a baking dish, and pour water into the dish, around tomatoes. Drizzle remaining $1/2$ tablespoon extra-virgin olive oil over each tomato.

9. Cover the baking dish with aluminum foil, and bake for 30 minutes.

10. Serve warm with tzatziki sauce.

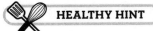 **HEALTHY HINT**

Bulgur wheat is a very easy wheat to prepare. It's also a great source of fiber and complex carbohydrates.

Vegetarian Stuffed Baked Potatoes

In this dish, tender potatoes are stuffed with a seasoned vegetable filling and baked in an earthy tomato sauce. You get plenty of fiber and protein, and the potatoes are filling without the need for any bread.

Yield:	Prep time:	Cook time:	Serving size:
6 potatoes	30 minutes	38 minutes	1 potato

Each serving has:			
408 calories	10g fat	1g saturated fat	9g protein
73g carbohydrates	9g dietary fiber	0mg cholesterol	1,054mg sodium

6 large potatoes, peeled	1 TB. seven spices
1 lb. baby spinach, chopped	1 (16-oz.) can plain tomato sauce
2 cups broccoli florets, finely chopped	1 TB. fresh thyme
1 large yellow onion, finely chopped	1 tsp. dried oregano
2 TB. minced garlic	1 tsp. ground black pepper
4 TB. extra-virgin olive oil	1/2 tsp. garlic powder
2 tsp. salt	

1. Preheat the oven to 450°F.

2. Trim bottom of potatoes so they stand on end. Cut off top quarter of potatoes, and set aside tops. Hollow out inside of potatoes, and stand potatoes in a large casserole dish. Finely chop potato flesh, and set aside.

3. In a large skillet over medium heat, cook spinach for 3 minutes.

4. Add broccoli, yellow onion, garlic, 2 tablespoons extra-virgin olive oil, 1 teaspoon salt, seven spices, and chopped potato flesh, and cook for 5 minutes.

5. Fill each potato with 3 tablespoons vegetable mixture, and place tops back on filled potatoes. Evenly drizzle remaining 2 tablespoons extra-virgin olive oil over potatoes, and bake for 15 minutes.

6. In a 2-quart pot over medium heat, combine tomato sauce, remaining 1 teaspoon salt, thyme, oregano, black pepper, and garlic powder, and simmer for 10 minutes.

7. After potatoes have baked for 15 minutes, add sauce mixture to the dish, and bake for 15 more minutes.

8. Remove from the oven, and serve warm.

Vegetarian Stuffed Squash

I love this dish because it's so easy to make and you really don't need any sides with it. The squash is filled with a combination of seasoned rice and vegetables and then cooked in a flavorful tomato sauce.

Yield:	Prep time:	Cook time:	Serving size:
8 stuffed zucchini	30 minutes	1 hour	1 stuffed zucchini

Each serving has:			
98 calories	1g fat	0g saturated fat	5g protein
20g carbohydrate	4g dietary fiber	0mg cholesterol	1,241mg sodium

8 (5-in.) light green zucchini	2 tsp. salt
1 cup long-grain rice, rinsed	1 tsp. ground black pepper
1 large tomato, finely diced	4 cups plain tomato sauce
1/2 large green bell pepper, ribs and seeds removed, and finely chopped	2 cups water
	1 tsp. dried mint
2 TB. minced garlic	

1. Trim off tops of zucchini, and hollow out zucchini. Set aside.

2. In a large bowl, combine long-grain rice, tomato, green bell pepper, 1 tablespoon garlic, 1 teaspoon salt, and 1/2 teaspoon black pepper.

3. Loosely stuff each zucchini with 3 or 4 tablespoons rice mixture. Do not overstuff.

4. In a large, 3-quart pot over low heat, combine tomato sauce, water, remaining 1 tablespoon garlic, remaining 1 teaspoon salt, remaining 1/2 teaspoon black pepper, and mint.

5. Add stuffed zucchini to tomato sauce, cover, and cook over low heat for 1 hour.

6. Serve warm.

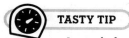 **TASTY TIP**

Instead of rice, you can use bulgur wheat (grind #2) as a healthy, flavorful alternative in the **Vegetarian Stuffed Squash** recipe.

Vegetarian Baked Spaghetti

This baked spaghetti combines tender noodles with bits of eggplant and a flavorful herb-seasoned sauce.

Yield:	Prep time:	Cook time:	Serving size:
10 cups	20 minutes	$1^1/_2$ hours	1 cup

Each serving has:			
310 calories	9g fat	2g saturated fat	11g protein
48g carbohydrate	5g dietary fiber	6mg cholesterol	965mg sodium

1 medium eggplant, diced

1 large white onion, finely chopped

1 medium green bell pepper, ribs and seeds removed, and finely chopped

2 TB. minced garlic

4 TB. extra-virgin olive oil

2 (16-oz.) can plain tomato sauce

1 (16-oz.) can diced tomatoes, with juice

3 TB. tomato paste

2 cups water

2 TB. sugar

$2^1/_2$ tsp. salt

1 tsp. dried oregano

1 tsp. dried thyme

$^1/_3$ cup fresh basil, chopped

3 TB. fresh Italian parsley, chopped

$^1/_2$ tsp. crushed red pepper flakes

$^1/_2$ tsp. ground black pepper

1 lb. spaghetti

1 cup shredded mozzarella cheese

1. In a large, 3-quart pot over medium heat, brown eggplant for 5 minutes.

2. Stir in white onion, green bell pepper, garlic, and extra-virgin olive oil, and cook for 5 minutes.

3. Add tomato sauce, diced tomatoes with juice, tomato paste, water, sugar, $1^1/_2$ teaspoons salt, oregano, thyme, basil, Italian parsley, crushed red pepper flakes, and black pepper, and stir. Reduce heat to low, and cook for 20 minutes.

4. Bring a large pot of water to a boil over high heat, and boil remaining 1 teaspoon salt and spaghetti for 8 minutes.

5. Preheat the oven to 450°F.

6. Drain spaghetti, pour into a large casserole dish, add pasta sauce, and toss to combine.

7. Cover dish with a piece of aluminum foil, and bake for 20 minutes.

8. Remove casserole dish from the oven, remove the foil, and sprinkle mozzarella cheese over spaghetti. Bake for 15 more minutes.

9. Remove spaghetti from the oven and let rest for 10 minutes before serving.

Vegetarian Potato Kibbeh

This vegetarian kibbeh uses potatoes as the binder for the bulgur wheat instead of meat. When combined with spices and a seasoned vegetable stuffing, it's delicious.

Yield:	Prep time:	Cook time:	Serving size:
1 (8×8-inch) casserole	40 minutes	40 minutes	$^1/_6$ of casserole

Each serving has:			
473 calories	33g fat	4g saturated fat	7g protein
40g carbohydrate	6g dietary fiber	0mg cholesterol	979mg sodium

1 cup bulgur wheat, grind #1	$^1/_2$ tsp. cayenne
1 cup warm water	1 tsp. ground black pepper
4 large boiled potatoes, peeled	$^1/_4$ cup plus 2 TB. extra-virgin olive oil
$^1/_2$ cup all-purpose flour	
$2^1/_2$ tsp. salt	$^1/_2$ medium red bell pepper
$^1/_2$ tsp. allspice	$^1/_2$ medium green bell pepper
$^1/_2$ tsp. cumin	$^1/_2$ medium yellow onion
$^1/_2$ tsp. ground coriander	$^1/_2$ cup pine nuts
$^1/_2$ tsp. ground nutmeg	$^1/_2$ cup walnuts
$^1/_2$ tsp. ground cloves	1 tsp. seven spices
$^1/_2$ tsp. ground cinnamon	1 tsp. sumac

1. In a large bowl, combine bulgur wheat and warm water, and set aside for 20 minutes.

2. Add potatoes, all-purpose flour, 2 teaspoons salt, allspice, cumin, coriander, nutmeg, cloves, cinnamon, cayenne, and black pepper, and knead together for about 4 or 5 minutes until well combined. Set aside.

3. In a medium skillet over medium heat, heat $^1/_4$ cup extra-virgin olive oil. Add red bell pepper, green bell pepper, and onions, and cook for 5 minutes.

4. Stir in remaining $^1/_2$ teaspoon salt, pine nuts, walnuts, seven spices, and sumac, and cook for 3 minutes.

5. Preheat the oven to 450°F. Grease an 8×8-inch baking dish with extra-virgin olive oil.

6. Divide kibbeh dough in half, and spread a layer of kibbeh dough on the bottom of the baking dish. Add a layer of sautéed vegetables and top with another layer of kibbeh dough.

7. Paint top of kibbeh with remaining 2 tablespoons extra-virgin olive oil, and cut kibbeh into 6 equal pieces. Bake for 30 minutes.

8. Let kibbeh rest for 15 minutes before serving.

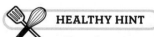 **HEALTHY HINT**

If you have an aversion to nuts, you can omit the walnuts and pine nuts from this dish.

Vegetarian Cabbage Rolls

Here, cabbage leaves are stuffed with a seasoned vegetable and rice mixture and cooked in a mild garlic tomato sauce.

Yield:	Prep time:	Cook time:	Serving size:
24 rolls	40 minutes	1$^1/_2$ hours	2 rolls

Each serving has:			
71 calories	0g fat	0g saturated fat	3g protein
16g carbohydrates	4g dietary fiber	0mg cholesterol	827mg sodium

1 large head green cabbage	1 tsp. ground black pepper
1 cup long-grain rice, rinsed	4 cups plain tomato sauce
2 medium zucchini, finely diced	2 cups water
4 TB. minced garlic	1 tsp. dried mint
2 tsp. salt	

1. Cut around core of cabbage with a knife, and remove core. Place cabbage, core side down, in a large, 3-quart pot. Cover cabbage with water, set over high heat, and cook for 30 minutes. Drain cabbage, set aside to cool, and separate leaves. (You need 24 leaves.)

2. In a large bowl, combine long-grain rice, zucchini, 1 tablespoon garlic, 1 teaspoon salt, and $^1/_2$ teaspoon black pepper.

3. In a 2-quart pot, combine tomato sauce, water, remaining 3 tablespoons garlic, mint, remaining 1 teaspoon salt, and remaining $^1/_2$ teaspoon black pepper.

4. Lay each cabbage leaf flat on your work surface, spoon 2 tablespoons filling on each leaf, and roll leaf. Layer rolls in a large pot, pour sauce into the pot, cover, and cook over medium-low heat for 1 hour.

5. Let rolls rest for 20 minutes before serving warm with Greek yogurt.

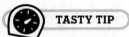

TASTY TIP

If the cabbage leaves are too big, you can cut them in half and make 2 rolls from 1 leaf.

Sensational Side Dishes

Side dishes accompany and complement main dishes. They're what make the main dish complete. And the good thing about sides is that you have countless choices for what can be a side dish. In this chapter, you explore some side dish ideas that can make your star dish really shine.

But can the supporting side dish steal the spotlight? Yes it can! Sometimes the side is so good it outshines the main dish. Whether it's rice, potatoes, beans, greens, or pasta, any side dish can be transformed into a star by using spices, herbs, fruits, and vegetables.

And why not have a full dinner of side dishes? They're just as healthy as main dishes and have just as much flavor. The next time you don't know what to cook, take a look at your side dish options, and make them the star of the show.

In This Chapter

- Rich and filling rice dishes
- Versatile veggie sides
- Transforming sides into main dishes

Brown Rice with Vermicelli Noodles

This is a nice twist on plain brown rice. The toasted noodles add a pleasing, toasted flavor to the earthy brown rice.

Yield:	Prep time:	Cook time:	Serving size:
2$^1/_2$ cups	20 minutes	45 minutes	$^1/_2$ cup

Each serving has:			
142 calories	9g fat	1g saturated fat	1g protein
15g carbohydrate	1g dietary fiber	0mg cholesterol	522mg sodium

3 TB. extra-virgin olive oil

$^1/_4$ cup vermicelli noodles

1 vegetable bouillon

2$^1/_4$ cups water

1 cup brown basmati rice

$^3/_4$ tsp. salt

1. Heat a 2-quart saucepan over low heat. Add extra-virgin olive oil and vermicelli noodles, and brown, stirring constantly, for 1 minute.

2. Add vegetable bouillon and water, and bring to a simmer.

3. When water comes to a simmer, add brown basmati rice and salt, and stir. Reduce heat to low, cover, and cook for 40 minutes.

4. After 40 minutes, turn off heat. Fluff rice with a fork, cover, and let rice sit for 15 to 20 minutes.

5. Serve warm.

 TASTY TIP

If you don't have or don't want to use bouillon, you can replace it and the water with 2$^1/_4$ cups vegetable broth or chicken broth instead. I love using chicken broth when I have it on hand.

Spicy Herb Potatoes (*Batata Harra*)

I try not to make these potatoes very often because I end up eating half of the plate by myself! These potatoes are baked until slightly crunchy and seasoned with garlic, fresh cilantro, and cayenne. The blend of herbs and spices adds a nice flavor kick.

Yield:	Prep time:	Cook time:	Serving size:
5 cups	20 minutes	25 minutes	1 cup
Each serving has:			
477 calories	12g fat	2g saturated fat	10g protein
83g carbohydrate	8g dietary fiber	0mg cholesterol	517mg sodium

15 small new red potatoes (1$\frac{1}{2}$ lb.), scrubbed and dried

1 tsp. salt

4 TB. extra-virgin olive oil

3 TB. minced garlic

1 cup fresh cilantro, finely chopped

$\frac{1}{2}$ tsp. cayenne

$\frac{1}{2}$ tsp. black pepper

1. Preheat the oven to 425°F.

2. Cut red potatoes into 1-inch pieces. Add potatoes to a large bowl, and toss with salt and 3 tablespoons extra-virgin olive oil.

3. Spread potatoes in an even layer on a baking sheet, and bake for 20 to 25 minutes or until golden. Remove from the oven, and let stand for 5 minutes.

4. Using a spatula, transfer potatoes to a large serving bowl.

5. Heat a small saucepan over low heat. Add remaining 1 tablespoon extra-virgin olive oil and garlic, and sauté for 3 minutes. Add garlic to potatoes.

6. Add cilantro, cayenne, and black pepper to potatoes, and gently toss to combine.

7. Serve warm or at room temperature.

MEDITERRANEAN MORSEL

Sometimes, if I don't have cilantro on hand, I like to use whatever fresh herbs are in my garden, like sage or rosemary. Try replacing the cilantro in this recipe with an herb you prefer.

Green Fava Beans

I make this dish a lot during the summer, when I can find fresh fava beans. I love how the garlic, cilantro, and lemon give the beans a huge flavor kick and make this dish irresistible.

Yield:	Prep time:	Cook time:	Serving size:
6 cups	20 minutes	30 minutes	1 cup

Each serving has:			
293 calories	8g fat	1g saturated fat	17g protein
41g carbohydrate	16g dietary fiber	0mg cholesterol	400mg sodium

3 TB. extra-virgin olive oil

1 large yellow onion, chopped

1 tsp. salt

8 cups fresh green fava beans (2 lb.)

3 TB. minced garlic

2 cups fresh cilantro, finely chopped

1 large lemon, cut in $^1/_2$

1. In a large, deep, skillet over medium heat, heat extra-virgin olive oil. Add yellow onion and $^1/_2$ teaspoon salt, and sauté for 5 minutes.

2. Wash and dry fava beans. Cut off stems, pull down to remove stringy veins, and repeat on other side. Chop bean pod into $^1/_2$-inch pieces.

3. Add fava beans to onions, and toss. Reduce heat to low, cover, and cook for 20 minutes, stirring every 5 minutes.

4. Add remaining $^1/_2$ teaspoon salt, garlic, and cilantro, and toss to combine. Cook, uncovered, for 5 minutes.

5. Spoon beans onto a plate, and squeeze $^1/_2$ of lemon over beans.

6. Serve with remaining lemon half on the side.

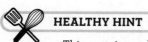 **HEALTHY HINT**

This protein- and fiber-rich dish goes great with brown rice and can become an entire meal on its own.

Yellow Rice

This rice is served very often in Middle Eastern restaurants, and I just love it alongside kabobs. The exotic taste of the saffron with the fluffy basmati rice is a great accompaniment to any main dish.

Yield:	Prep time:	Cook time:	Serving size:
4 cups	5 minutes	40 minutes	1 cup

Each serving has:			
168 calories	7g fat	1g saturated fat	2g protein
22g carbohydrate	0g dietary fiber	0mg cholesterol	768mg sodium

4 cups water	2 cups basmati rice
1 chicken or vegetable bouillon	2 TB. extra-virgin olive oil
$^1/_2$ tsp. or 10 strands saffron	1 tsp. salt

1. In a 2-quart saucepan over medium heat, bring water, chicken bouillon, and saffron strands to a simmer.

2. Add basmati rice, extra-virgin olive oil, and salt, reduce heat to low, and bring to a simmer over low heat. Cover and cook for 40 minutes.

3. After 40 minutes, remove from heat. Fluff rice with a fork, cover, and let rice stand for 20 minutes.

4. Serve warm.

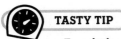 **TASTY TIP**

For a little more flavor and color, add $^1/_2$ teaspoon turmeric to the rice as it cooks.

Pickled Persian Cucumbers

These cucumbers are often served with falafel and shawarma. They're crunchy and tangy with a hint of garlic—the perfect accompaniment to any sandwich.

Yield:	Prep time:	Serving size:	
10 pickles	10 minutes	1 pickle	
Each serving has:			
55 calories	0g fat	0g saturated fat	2g protein
11g carbohydrate	2g dietary fiber	0mg cholesterol	1,402mg sodium

10 medium Persian cucumbers	2 cups white vinegar
2 cloves garlic, sliced	6 tsp. salt
2 cups water	

1. In a large jar, place Persian cucumbers and garlic.

2. In a large bowl, whisk together water, white vinegar, and salt until salt is dissolved.

3. Pour enough of vinegar mixture into the jar to fill to the top. Add the lid, seal the jar, gently shake to mix.

4. Let jar sit at room temperature for 1 week and then refrigerate.

5. Refrigerate pickles after opening.

Pickled Turnips (*Kabees*)

These sour and spicy pickled turnips have a beautiful fuchsia color, thanks to the beets.

Yield:	Prep time:	Serving size:	
4 cups	10 minutes	$^1/_3$ cup	
Each serving has:			
18 calories	0g fat	0g saturated fat	0g protein
3g carbohydrate	1g dietary fiber	0mg cholesterol	608mg sodium

3 large turnips, peeled and cut into $^1/_4$-in. slices	$^1/_2$ medium jalapeño, sliced
1 large beet, peeled and cut into $^1/_4$-in. slices	$1^1/_2$ cups water
2 cloves garlic, sliced	$1^1/_2$ cups white vinegar
	3 tsp. salt

1. In a large jar, place turnips, beets, garlic, and jalapeño.

2. In a large bowl, whisk together water, white vinegar, and salt until salt is dissolved.

3. Pour enough of vinegar mixture into the jar to fill to the top. Add the lid, seal the jar, and gently shake to mix.

4. Store the jar in the refrigerator for 1 week.

5. Refrigerate after opening.

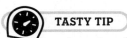 **TASTY TIP**

> If you don't like spicy food, you can omit the jalapeño from this recipe.

Dandelion Greens

My mom used to make me eat these greens when I was a kid because they were filled with iron and nutrients. The green flavor of the dandelion leaves is cut by the sweetness of the onions and the citrus of the fresh lemon juice.

Yield:	Prep time:	Cook time:	Serving size:
6 cups	15 minutes	50 minutes	1 cup

Each serving has:			
218 calories	18g fat	3g saturated fat	2g protein
13g carbohydrate	3g dietary fiber	0mg cholesterol	1,001mg sodium

4 cups dandelion greens (2 lb.)	$^1/_2$ cup extra-virgin olive oil
14 cups water	4 large white onions, sliced
$2^1/_2$ tsp. salt	1 large lemon, cut into quarters

1. Thoroughly wash dandelion greens in a large bowl of water three times to remove any dirt, discarding water after each wash. Chop greens into 1-inch pieces.

2. In a large pot over medium-high heat, bring water to a simmer. Add 1 teaspoon salt and dandelion greens, and simmer, stirring occasionally, for 20 minutes. Drain greens, and squeeze out any excess water.

3. Preheat a large skillet over medium heat. Add $^1/_4$ cup extra-virgin olive oil and $^1/_2$ of white onions, and cook, stirring occasionally, for 5 minutes.

4. Add dandelion greens and 1 teaspoon salt to the skillet, reduce heat to low, and cook for 15 more minutes.

5. Transfer dandelion mixture to a serving plate.

6. In the skillet, heat remaining $^1/_4$ cup extra-virgin olive oil. Add remaining $^1/_2$ teaspoon salt and $^1/_2$ of remaining onions, and cook, stirring occasionally, for 20 minutes or until lightly browned.

7. Top dandelion greens with browned onions, squeeze juice of $^1/_2$ lemon on top, and serve with 2 remaining lemon quarters.

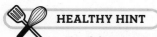 **HEALTHY HINT**

> Dandelion greens have many health benefits. They are filled with iron, antioxidants, calcium, and even protein.

Spiced Meat and Rice

I loved when my mom made this dish. I would start eating it before she could carry the bowl to the table. The browned meat with the seasoned rice make this dish hearty and filling.

Yield:	Prep time:	Cook time:	Serving size:
5 cups	5 minutes	47 minutes	1 cup

Each serving has:			
191 calories	8g fat	2g saturated fat	10g protein
19g carbohydrate	1g dietary fiber	27mg cholesterol	726mg sodium

$^1/_2$ lb. ground beef

2 cups long-grain rice, rinsed

4 cups water

1 tsp. seven spices

$^1/_2$ tsp. cinnamon

$1^1/_2$ tsp. salt

1 TB. extra-virgin olive oil

1. In a 2-quart pot over medium heat, brown beef for 5 minutes, breaking up chunks with a wooden spoon.

2. Add long-grain rice, stir, and cook for 2 minutes.

3. Add water, seven spices, cinnamon, salt, and extra-virgin olive oil, and stir. Bring to a simmer, cover, reduce heat to low, and cook for 40 minutes.

4. Remove from heat, fluff rice with a fork, cover, and let the rice stand for 10 more minutes.

5. Serve warm.

Sautéed Zucchini and Mushrooms

I serve this veggie sauté as an accompaniment to any protein, fish, chicken, or steak main dish. The thyme lends its zesty lemon flavor to brighten up the earthiness of the zucchini and mushrooms.

Yield:	Prep time:	Cook time:	Serving size:
4 cups	10 minutes	12 minutes	1 cup

Each serving has:			
126 calories	11g fat	2g saturated fat	3g protein
6g carbohydrate	2g dietary fiber	0mg cholesterol	592mg sodium

3 TB. extra-virgin olive oil

1 large white onion, chopped

2 cups crimini mushrooms, rinsed and chopped

1 tsp. salt

1 TB. minced garlic

2 medium zucchini, chopped

2 TB. fresh thyme

$^1/_2$ tsp. ground black pepper

1. In a large skillet over medium heat, heat extra-virgin olive oil. Add white onion, crimini mushrooms, and salt, and toss. Cook for 5 minutes.

2. Stir in garlic, and cook for another 2 minutes.

3. Add zucchini, thyme, and black pepper, and stir to combine. Cook for 5 minutes.

4. Serve warm.

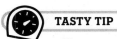 **TASTY TIP**

You can use any other vegetables related to zucchini, like pumpkin or squash, in this recipe. Try your favorite zucchini, for example.

Delectable Desserts

Yes, you can have dessert on the Mediterranean diet, but you must remember to indulge in *moderation*. Desserts can add a lot of calories to your day, but having up to three bites of dessert is a great way to satisfy your craving and control your calories at the same time.

The Mediterranean desserts in Part 6 incorporate many different varieties of fruit and nuts—both of which are very healthy and taste great separate or combined in a recipe. I also share cookies, cakes, and other tempting treats you'll love serving at the end of Mediterranean meals.

CHAPTER 19

Cookies, Baklava, and More

Sweets are the perfect closing to a delicious meal. But it's very easy to pass on this part of the meal because of the abundance of calories these little bites contain. But you don't have to anymore.

You can fit sweets in your Mediterranean diet plan. Remember, though, that desserts are at the top of the Mediterranean diet pyramid, indicating you should eat them sparingly. But that shouldn't be a problem because with the balance of nutrients you'll be getting from your meals, your sugar cravings should be minimal. A good way to work desserts into your diet is to try to assign a day of the week when you can have desserts, maybe during the weekend or the night your favorite show is on.

Baklava, popular in the Mediterranean, is one of the oldest desserts in the world. Different versions layer different ingredients between the flaky phyllo dough, but traditionally, nuts are the ingredient of choice. You'll also see that fruits are prevalent in Mediterranean desserts because they're so readily available.

In This Chapter

- Crave-worthy cookies
- Sweet and flaky baklava
- Desserts on the Mediterranean diet

Pistachio Cookies

Talk about small bites of happiness. These slightly sweet butter cookies are bursting with the nuttiness of ground pistachios.

Yield:	Prep time:	Cook time:	Serving size:
36 cookies	$1^1/_2$ hours	12 minutes	1 cookie

Each serving has:			
115 calories	7g fat	3g saturated fat	2g protein
12g carbohydrate	1g dietary fiber	19mg cholesterol	71mg sodium

1 cup butter, at room temperature	1 cup pistachios, ground
1 cup sugar	1 tsp. baking powder
1 large egg	$^1/_2$ tsp. salt
2 tsp. vanilla extract or flavoring	2 TB. confectioners' sugar
2 cups all-purpose flour	

1. In a blender, cream together butter and sugar for about 2 minutes.

2. Beat in egg and vanilla extract for about 30 seconds.

3. Blend in all-purpose flour, pistachios, baking powder, and salt until well combined.

4. Spoon dough onto a sheet of plastic wrap. Using the plastic wrap, form dough into a $1^1/_2$-inch log, and refrigerate for 1 hour.

5. Preheat the oven to 375°F. Line a baking sheet with parchment paper.

6. Cut log into about 36 ($^1/_8$-inch) slices, and place slices 1 inch apart on the prepared baking sheet.

7. Bake for 12 minutes or until edges start to turn slightly golden brown.

8. Let cookies cool on the baking sheet for 5 to 10 minutes, dust with confectioners' sugar, and serve.

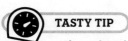 **TASTY TIP**

If you don't like pistachios, feel free to use another nut like walnuts, pecans, or macadamia nuts.

Date Cookies

These dainty cookies are subtle and sweet but can still satisfy your sweet tooth and be served at tea time.

Yield:	Prep time:	Cook time:	Serving size:
18 cookies	1¹/₂ hours	15 minutes	1 cookie
Each serving has:			
212 calories	10g fat	2g saturated fat	3g protein
29g carbohydrate	2g dietary fiber	17mg cholesterol	85mg sodium

2¹/₂ cups all-purpose flour	¹/₂ cup vegetable oil
¹/₂ tsp. salt	¹/₂ cup warm water
1 TB. baking powder	10 dates, pitted
2 tsp. active dry yeast	3 TB. butter, at room temperature
3 TB. sugar	1 large egg, beaten
1 tsp. ground cinnamon	¹/₄ cup sesame seeds

1. In a large bowl, combine all-purpose flour, salt, baking powder, yeast, sugar, ¹/₂ teaspoon cinnamon, vegetable oil, and warm water, and knead for 3 minutes. Cover and set aside for 1 hour.

2. Preheat the oven to 350°F.

3. In a food processor fitted with a chopping blade, blend dates, butter, and remaining ¹/₂ teaspoon cinnamon for 30 seconds.

4. Dust your work surface with flour, place dough on the surface, and knead 10 times. Roll dough into a 16-inch oval.

5. Spoon date mixture along length of oval, and roll dough into a 16-inch-long log. Brush log with beaten egg, and sprinkle with sesame seeds. Cut log into 18 equal-size pieces and place 1 inch apart on a baking sheet. Bake for 15 minutes.

6. Let cookies cool on the baking sheet for 5 to 10 minutes, and serve.

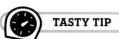 **TASTY TIP**

These dates are great for an afternoon tea. They're not too sweet and go great with the flavor of an Earl Grey tea.

Holiday Date Cookies (*Maamoul*)

These traditional buttery holiday cookies are filled with an earthy walnut or date filling and then dusted with confectioners' sugar.

Yield:	Prep time:	Cook time:	Serving size:
24 cookies	50 minutes	20 minutes	1 cookie

Each serving has:			
208 calories	11g fat	5g saturated fat	3g protein
25g carbohydrate	2g dietary fiber	21mg cholesterol	105mg sodium

1¹/₂ cups all-purpose flour	1¹/₂ cups ground walnuts
1¹/₂ cups semolina flour	¹/₄ cup sugar
1 tsp. baking powder	¹/₄ tsp. ground cinnamon
¹/₂ tsp. salt	10 dates, pitted
1 cup butter, melted	1 TB. water
¹/₄ cup whole milk	3 TB. confectioners' sugar
1 TB. orange blossom water	

1. In a large bowl, combine all-purpose flour, semolina flour, baking powder, salt, butter, whole milk, and 1 tablespoon orange blossom water. Cover with plastic wrap, and set aside for 30 minutes.

2. Preheat the oven to 400°F.

3. In a food processor fitted with a chopping blade, blend walnuts, sugar, and cinnamon for 30 seconds. Transfer to a bowl, and set aside.

4. In the food processor, blend dates, orange blossom water, and water for 30 seconds or until smooth.

5. Pinch off 3 tablespoons of dough, and using your hands, flatten dough into a 3-inch circle. Place 1 tablespoon either walnut mixture or date mixture in center of dough circle, and seal dough around filling, forming a ball.

6. Press ball into a cookie mold or create a design on surface of dough using the back of a fork.

7. Place cookie on a baking sheet, repeat with remaining dough and filling, and bake for 20 minutes.

8. Cool cookies on a cooling rack for 20 minutes.

9. Dust cookies with confectioners' sugar, and serve.

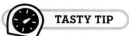 **TASTY TIP**

If you don't have or cannot find orange blossom water, replace that flavoring with the flavoring of your choice—vanilla extract, almond extract, coconut extract, etc.

Chocolate-Dipped Pistachio Sugar Cookies

This sugar cookie is full of Mediterranean flavors. It's simply amazing.

Yield:	Prep time:	Cook time:	Serving size:
36 cookies	1¹/₂ hours	12 minutes	1 cookie

Each serving has:			
184 calories	11g fat	6g saturated fat	3g protein
19g carbohydrate	1g dietary fiber	32mg cholesterol	82mg sodium

1 cup butter, at room temperature	1 tsp. baking powder
1 cup sugar	¹/₂ tsp. salt
2 large eggs	2 cups milk chocolate chips
1 TB. vanilla extract	¹/₂ cup heavy cream
2¹/₂ cups all-purpose flour	1 cup pistachios, finely chopped

1. In a blender, cream together butter and sugar for about 2 minutes.

2. Beat in eggs and vanilla extract for about 30 seconds.

3. Stir in all-purpose flour, baking powder, and salt until well combined.

4. Transfer dough to a sheet of plastic wrap. Using the plastic wrap, form dough into a 3×12-inch flat rectangle, and refrigerate for 1 hour.

5. Preheat the oven to 375°F. Line a baking sheet with parchment paper.

6. Cut dough log into about 36 (¹/₃-inch) slices. Place slices 1 inch apart on the prepared baking sheet. Bake for 12 minutes or until edges start to turn slightly golden brown.

7. Cool cookies for 15 minutes.

8. In a medium bowl, combine milk chocolate chips and heavy cream. Using a double boiler or a microwave, melt chocolate, stirring intermittently until melted.

9. Dip half of each cookie in chocolate, and roll chocolate-dipped part of cookie in pistachios. Place cookies on a piece of parchment paper and allow chocolate to firm up.

Jam Cookies

These delightful little shortbread cookie sandwiches with a spoonful of jam in the center bring back memories of my childhood, when my mother used to make them and she'd let me spread the jam on each cookie.

Yield:	Prep time:	Cook time:	Serving size:
24 cookie sandwiches	1 hour	15 minutes	1 cookie sandwich

Each serving has:			
270 calories	12g fat	7g saturated fat	2g protein
40g carbohydrate	1g dietary fiber	31mg cholesterol	141mg sodium

1$^1/_2$ cups butter, at room temperature	$^1/_2$ tsp. salt
1 cup sugar	2 cups apricot jam
1 TB. vanilla extract	3 TB. confectioners' sugar
3$^1/_2$ cups all-purpose flour	

1. Using a blender, cream together butter and sugar for about 2 minutes.

2. Beat in vanilla extract for about 30 seconds.

3. Stir in 3 cups all-purpose flour and salt, until well combined.

4. Transfer dough to a sheet of plastic wrap. Using the plastic wrap, form dough into disc. Refrigerate for 30 minutes.

5. Preheat the oven to 400°F. Line a baking sheet with parchment paper.

6. Dust your work surface with some flour, and roll out discs to $^1/_8$ inch thickness. Using a 1-inch star cookie cutter, cut out 48 stars from cookie dough. Place cookies 1 inch apart on the prepared baking sheet, and bake for 15 minutes or until edges start to slightly turn golden brown.

7. Cook cookies on a cooling rack for about 20 minutes.

8. Spread 1 or 2 tablespoons apricot jam on 24 cookies, and place remaining 24 cookies on top of jam cookies to form sandwiches. Dust cookies with confectioners' sugar, and serve.

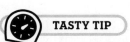 **TASTY TIP**

Instead of apricot jam, you can use whatever flavor of jam you like or is in season.

Baklava

Baklava, made with layers of flaky phyllo dough stuffed with a sweet nutty filling, is a very traditional Mediterranean dessert.

Yield:	Prep time:	Cook time:	Serving size:
12 pieces	2¹/₂ hours	31 minutes	1 piece
Each serving has:			
311 calories	16g fat	6g saturated fat	4g protein
38g carbohydrate	2g dietary fiber	20mg cholesterol	295 mg sodium

1 cup walnuts	25 (8×8-in.) sheets phyllo dough
¹/₂ tsp. ground cinnamon	¹/₂ cup butter, melted
¹/₂ tsp. ground nutmeg	1 cup Simple Syrup (recipe in Chapter 21), at room temperature
¹/₄ cup sugar	
¹/₄ tsp. salt	

1. Preheat the oven to 350°F.

2. In a food processor fitted with a chopping blade, blend walnuts, cinnamon, nutmeg, sugar, and salt for 30 seconds.

3. In an 8×8-inch pan, begin to layer phyllo dough. Add 10 sheets, buttering each sheet as you lay it in the pan. Then sprinkle phyllo dough with ¹/₂ of nut mixture. Layer next 5 phyllo sheets, brushing each sheet with butter. Sprinkle rest of nut mixture over top, and add remaining 10 layers of phyllo, again brushing each sheet with butter.

4. Using a sharp knife, cut baklava into 12 equal pieces. Bake for 20 to 25 minutes or until phyllo turns golden brown.

5. Pour Simple Syrup over baklava, and let it soak for at least 2 hours before serving.

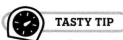 **TASTY TIP**

> If you don't like walnuts, you definitely don't have to use them in this recipe. Almonds, pine nuts, pistachios, and even peanuts are all great alternatives in baklava.

Chocolate-Peanut Baklava

This is a twist on the traditional baklava. This rich version is filled with peanuts and melted chocolate—almost like a candy bar but with a flaky crust.

Yield:	Prep time:	Cook time:	Serving size:
12 pieces	2^1/$_2$ hours	31 minutes	1 piece

Each serving has:			
280 calories	15g fat	7g saturated fat	5g protein
32g carbohydrate	2g dietary fiber	22mg cholesterol	252mg sodium

^{1}/$_2$ cup milk chocolate chips

^{1}/$_2$ cup peanuts, chopped

25 (8×8-in.) sheets phyllo dough

^{1}/$_2$ cup butter, melted

^{1}/$_2$ cup Simple Syrup (recipe in Chapter 21), at room temperature

1. Preheat the oven to 350°F.

2. In a medium bowl, combine milk chocolate chips and peanuts.

3. In an 8×8-inch pan, begin to layer phyllo dough. Add 10 sheets, buttering each sheet as you lay it in the pan. Then sprinkle phyllo dough with ^{1}/$_2$ chocolate-peanut mixture. Layer next 5 phyllo sheets, brushing each sheet with butter. Sprinkle rest of chocolate-peanut mixture over top, and add remaining 10 layers of phyllo, again brushing each sheet with butter.

4. Using a sharp knife, cut baklava into 12 equal pieces. Bake for 20 to 25 minutes or until phyllo turns golden brown.

5. Pour Simple Syrup over baklava, and let it soak for at least 2 hours before serving.

Date Balls

These bite-size date treats are naturally sweet with a nice, toasted nutty flavor, thanks to the walnuts.

Yield:	Prep time:	Cook time:	Serving size:
16 date balls	10 minutes	5 minutes	1 date ball
Each serving has:			
209 calories	15g fat	6g saturated fat	4g protein
19g carbohydrate	3g dietary fiber	15mg cholesterol	56mg sodium

$^3/_4$ cup walnuts

12 medjool dates, pitted

$^1/_2$ cup butter, melted

1 cup pistachios, ground

1 cup coconut flakes

1. Preheat the oven to 450°F.

2. Evenly spread walnuts on a baking sheet, and toast for 5 minutes.

3. In a food processor fitted with a chopping blade, blend toasted walnuts for 30 seconds or until evenly ground. Transfer walnuts to a medium bowl.

4. In the food processor, blend medjool dates and butter for 2 minutes until mixture resembles a paste.

5. Add date paste to ground walnuts, and mix to combine.

6. Place ground pistachios in a small bowl, and place coconut flakes in a separate small bowl.

7. Spray a bit of cooking spray on your hands, and spoon about 2 tablespoons date mixture into your hands and roll to form a ball. Immediately roll date ball into either ground pistachios or coconut flakes.

8. Place each date ball in a mini cupcake liner, and serve.

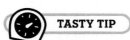 **TASTY TIP**

If you want the date balls to become a bit firmer, refrigerate them for 30 minutes before serving.

Fig Bars

Fig trees are abundant along the Mediterranean because the weather creates a perfect growing environment for them. The naturally sweet figs they produce are great for desserts.

Yield:	Prep time:	Cook time:	Serving size:
12 fig bars	1¹/₂ hours	30 minutes	1 fig bar

Each serving has:			
288 calories	14g fat	7g saturated fat	4g protein
38g carbohydrate	3g dietary fiber	28mg cholesterol	176mg sodium

¹/₂ cup plus 3 TB. butter, at room temperature

¹/₄ cup plus 2 TB. sugar

1 tsp. vanilla extract or flavoring

1¹/₄ cups all-purpose flour

1¹/₂ cups dried figs, chopped

1 cup hot water

¹/₂ cup walnuts

¹/₄ cup brown sugar, packed

¹/₂ cup instant oats

¹/₂ tsp. ground cinnamon

¹/₂ tsp. ground nutmeg

¹/₂ tsp. salt

1. In a medium bowl, and using an electric mixer on medium-high speed, cream together ¹/₂ cup butter, ¹/₄ cup sugar, and vanilla extract for 2 minutes.

2. Add 1 cup all-purpose flour, and blend for 30 seconds.

3. Place chopped figs in a small bowl, pour in hot water, and let them sit for 20 minutes.

4. Preheat the oven to 350°F.

5. Press dough into the bottom of a 9×9-inch pan, and bake for 10 minutes.

6. Add walnuts to figs, and mix well, slightly smashing with the back of a fork. Evenly distribute fig mixture over crust in the pan.

7. In a small bowl, combine remaining ¹/₄ cup flour, brown sugar, instant oats, cinnamon, nutmeg, and salt.

8. Using a pastry cutter or fork, cut remaining 3 tablespoons butter into oat mixture until you get a crumbly mixture. Spoon crumble topping over fig filling, and bake for 20 minutes.

9. Let bars cool for 1 hour before cutting and serving.

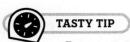 **TASTY TIP**

For a nuttier flavor, add ¹/₄ cup sesame seeds to the crumb topping.

Fig Puffs

This simple and easy dessert features crunchy puff pastry filled with oozing sweet figs and mascarpone cheese.

Yield:	Prep time:	Cook time:	Serving size:
6 fig puffs	30 minutes	15 minutes	1 fig puff

Each serving has:			
503 calories	33g fat	12g saturated fat	7g protein
48g carbohydrate	4g dietary fiber	48mg cholesterol	128mg sodium

12 dried figs, chopped

1 cup hot water

8 oz. mascarpone cheese

$^1/_2$ tsp. ground nutmeg

$^1/_2$ tsp. ground cinnamon

2 TB. honey

6 (4×4-in.) pieces puff pastry

$^1/_4$ cup whole milk

2 TB. sugar

1. In a medium bowl, combine figs and hot water. Let sit for 20 minutes. Drain any excess water from figs.

2. To figs, add mascarpone cheese, nutmeg, cinnamon, and honey, and stir to combine.

3. Lay out 1 piece of puff pastry, spoon 2 tablespoons fig mixture into center of puff pastry, and fold over one corner of pastry to the opposite corner, forming a triangle. Using a fork, press down along the side to seal pastry. Repeat with remaining pastry sheets and fig mixture.

4. Place pastries on a baking sheet, brush with whole milk, and sprinkle with sugar. Bake for 15 minutes or until golden brown.

5. Let pastries cool for 10 minutes before serving.

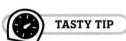 **TASTY TIP**

These also make terrific breakfast pastries.

Coconut Puffs (Macaroons)

These treats are more commonly known as coconut macaroons, but as a kid, I always called them coconut puffs. Whatever you call them, they're slightly sweet, crunchy on the outside, and chewy on the inside.

Yield:	Prep time:	Cook time:	Serving size:
24 macaroons	20 minutes	25 minutes	1 macaroon

Each serving has:			
154 calories	7g fat	6g saturated fat	3g protein
22g carbohydrate	2g dietary fiber	8mg cholesterol	107mg sodium

1 (14-oz.) can sweetened condensed milk

1 (14-oz.) bag sweetened coconut flakes

3 TB. all-purpose flour

1 TB. vanilla extract

3 large egg whites

$1/_4$ tsp. salt

1. Preheat the oven to 350°F. Line a baking sheet with parchment paper.

2. In a large bowl, combine sweetened condensed milk, sweetened coconut flakes, all-purpose flour, and vanilla extract.

3. In another large bowl, and using an electric mixer on high speed, blend egg whites and salt for about 4 minutes or until white peaks form.

4. In three batches, gently fold coconut mixture into beaten egg whites.

5. Spoon coconut mixture about 3 tablespoons at a time in mounds on the baking sheet about 2 inches apart. Bake for 25 minutes or until macaroons are golden brown.

6. Using a spatula, transfer macaroons to a flat surface to cool.

7. Serve at room temperature.

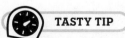 **TASTY TIP**

For extra decadence, drizzle the puffs with melted dark chocolate before serving.

Crave-Worthy Cakes

When you think of cake, maybe you think of layered chocolate or vanilla cakes with rich and creamy frostings. But that's not what cake is about in the Mediterranean. Mediterranean cakes have just as much flavor, but in a different way, flavored with syrups, jams, fruits, and spices and with an earthy, more natural taste—but they definitely satisfy any sweet tooth!

Mediterranean desserts also make use of olive oil and yogurt. Because olive oil is the fat of choice in the Mediterranean, it makes sense it would be used in dessert recipes. The trick is to use a *light* olive oil—one with fruity notes rather than a strong olive flavor—so your flavors won't clash.

Yogurt is used quite often in desserts and cakes to add moisture. The thickness and creaminess of the yogurt helps keep your cakes from drying out—and replaces a lot of the fat usually needed to do that job in other recipes.

In This Chapter

- Mouthwatering Mediterranean cakes
- Moist, yogurt-based cakes
- Delightful doughnuts
- Sweet and creamy cheesecake

Eggless Farina Cake (*Namoura*)

This thick and rich cake has a nice, nutty flavor thanks to the farina and semolina. Soaked with Simple Syrup, it's sweet, sticky, and delicious.

Yield:	Prep time:	Cook time:	Serving size:
1 (9×13-inch) cake; 15 pieces	1¹/₂ hours	40 minutes	1 piece

Each serving has:			
259 calories	12g fat	6g saturated fat	3g protein
37g carbohydrate	1g dietary fiber	27mg cholesterol	83mg sodium

2 cups farina	1 cup whole milk
¹/₂ cup *semolina*	³/₄ cup butter, melted
¹/₂ cup all-purpose flour	¹/₄ cup water
1 TB. baking powder	2 TB. tahini paste
1 tsp. active dry yeast	15 almonds
¹/₂ cup sugar	2 cups Simple Syrup (recipe in Chapter 21)
¹/₂ cup plain Greek yogurt	

1. In a large bowl, combine farina, semolina, all-purpose flour, baking powder, yeast, sugar, Greek yogurt, whole milk, butter, and water. Set aside for 15 minutes.

2. Preheat the oven to 375°F.

3. Spread tahini paste evenly in the bottom of a 9×13-inch baking pan, and pour in cake batter. Arrange almonds on top of batter, about where each slice will be. Bake for 45 minutes or until golden brown.

4. Remove cake from the oven, and using a toothpick, poke holes throughout cake for Simple Syrup to seep into. Pour syrup over cake, and let cake sit for 1 hour to absorb syrup.

5. Cool cake completely before cutting and serving.

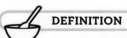 **DEFINITION**

Farina is a cereal food made from **semolina,** which is the by-product of the milling of durum wheat. Both are used to make baked goods, pastas, and cereal. They have a nutty flavor and add a nice texture to this cake.

Turmeric Cake (*Sfoof*)

This cake is light, fluffy, and just sweet enough. It has an amazing, distinct flavor thanks to the turmeric, but it's not overwhelming.

Yield:	Prep time:	Cook time:	Serving size:
1 (8×8-inch) cake; 12 pieces	15 minutes	27 minutes	1 piece

Each serving has:			
286 calories	16g fat	2g saturated fat	4g protein
34g carbohydrate	1g dietary fiber	1mg cholesterol	126mg sodium

$1^1/_2$ cups all-purpose flour	1 cup water
1 cup sugar	$^1/_2$ tsp. salt
1 TB. turmeric	1 TB. baking powder
$^3/_4$ cup vegetable oil	$^1/_4$ cup pine nuts
$^1/_2$ cup dry milk	

1. Preheat the oven to 425°F. Lightly coat an 8×8-inch baking pan with cooking spray, and dust the sides of the pan with about 2 tablespoons all-purpose flour.

2. In a large bowl, and using an electric mixer on medium speed, blend all-purpose flour, sugar, turmeric, vegetable oil, dry milk, water, salt, and baking powder for 2 minutes.

3. Pour batter into the prepared pan, and sprinkle pine nuts over top. Bake for 25 to 27 minutes or until a toothpick inserted in center of cake comes out dry.

4. Cool cake completely before cutting and serving.

Yogurt Cake

This dense lemon-flavored cake has a very light flavor. It's perfect for an afternoon treat.

Yield:	Prep time:	Cook time:	Serving size:
1 (9-inch round) cake; 12 pieces	15 minutes	55 minutes	1 piece

Each serving has:			
277 calories	10g fat	2g saturated fat	5g protein
42g carbohydrate	1g dietary fiber	36mg cholesterol	117mg sodium

1 cup plain Greek yogurt

1 cup sugar

2 large eggs

1 TB. vanilla extract

4 TB. fresh lemon juice

1 TB. lemon zest

$^1/_2$ cup vegetable or light olive oil

$1^3/_4$ cups all-purpose flour

2 tsp. baking powder

$^1/_2$ tsp. salt

1 cup confectioners' sugar

1. Preheat the oven to 350°F. Lightly coat a 9-inch-round cake pan with cooking spray, and dust the pan using about 2 tablespoons all-purpose flour.

2. In a large bowl, using an electric mixer on medium speed, blend Greek yogurt, sugar, eggs, vanilla extract, 2 tablespoons lemon juice, lemon zest, and vegetable oil for about 2 minutes.

3. Add all-purpose flour, baking powder, and salt, and blend for 2 more minutes.

4. Pour batter into the prepared cake pan, and bake for 55 minutes or until a toothpick inserted in center of cake comes out clean. Cool cake completely.

5. In a small bowl, whisk together confectioners' sugar and remaining 2 tablespoons lemon juice to make glaze.

6. When cake is cool, pour glaze over top, cut, and serve.

Date Cake

This is a sweet, sticky date cake with a nutty tahini sauce on top that complements the sweetness of the dates. It's indulgent and satisfying.

Yield:	Prep time:	Cook time:	Serving size:
1 (9×13-inch) cake; 16 pieces	30 minutes	35 minutes	1 piece

Each serving has:			
242 calories	8g fat	4g saturated fat	4g protein
41g carbohydrate	2g dietary fiber	42mg cholesterol	204mg sodium

8 dates, pitted and finely chopped	$2^1/_2$ cups all-purpose flour
$^3/_4$ cup water	$^1/_2$ tsp. salt
1 tsp. baking soda	$^1/_2$ tsp. cinnamon
$^3/_4$ cup sugar	2 tsp. baking powder
$^1/_2$ cup butter	$^3/_4$ cup confectioners' sugar
2 large eggs	3 TB. whole milk
1 TB. vanilla extract	2 TB. tahini paste

1. Preheat the oven to 350°F. Lightly coat a 9×13-inch cake pan or Bundt pan with cooking spray, and dust with about 2 tablespoons all-purpose flour.

2. In a medium saucepan over low heat, combine dates and water, and cook, stirring occasionally, for 5 minutes. Remove from heat.

3. Stir in baking soda, remove date mixture from the pan, and set aside to cool.

4. In a large bowl, and using an electric mixer on medium speed, blend cooled dates, sugar, butter, eggs, and vanilla extract for 2 minutes.

5. Add all-purpose flour, salt, cinnamon, and baking powder, blend for 2 more minutes.

6. Pour batter into the prepared pan, and bake for 35 minutes.

7. Cool cake completely.

8. In a small bowl, whisk together confectioners' sugar, whole milk, and tahini paste. If mixture is too thick, add another 1 tablespoon milk until it has the consistency of glaze.

9. When cake is cool, pour glaze over top, cut, and serve.

Olive Oil Cake

This cake has earthy undertones with a slight tang from the cranberries and oranges.

Yield:	Prep time:	Cook time:	Serving size:
1 (9-inch-round) cake; 14 pieces	15 minutes	45 minutes	1 piece

Each serving has:			
218 calories	9g fat	1g saturated fat	4g protein
31g carbohydrate	1g dietary fiber	31mg cholesterol	146mg sodium

2 large eggs	1^3/$_4$ cups all-purpose flour
^{3}/$_4$ cup sugar	^{1}/$_2$ tsp. salt
^{1}/$_2$ cup light olive oil	2 tsp. baking powder
1 cup plain Greek yogurt	^{1}/$_2$ tsp. baking soda
3 TB. fresh orange juice	^{3}/$_4$ cup dried cranberries
2 TB. orange zest	2 TB. confectioners' sugar

1. Preheat the oven to 350°F. Lightly coat a 9-inch-round cake pan or Bundt pan with cooking spray, and dust with about 2 tablespoons all-purpose flour.

2. In a large bowl, and using an electric mixer on medium speed, blend eggs and sugar for 2 minutes.

3. Blend in light olive oil, Greek yogurt, orange juice, and orange zest for 2 more minutes.

4. Add all-purpose flour, salt, baking powder, and baking soda and blend for 1 more minute.

5. Using a spatula or wooden spoon, fold cranberries into batter.

6. Pour batter into the prepared pan, and bake for 45 minutes or until a toothpick inserted in center of cake comes out clean.

7. Cool cake completely.

8. Dust top of cake with confectioners' sugar, cut, and serve.

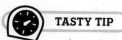 **TASTY TIP**

If you don't like dried cranberries, you can substitute golden raisins or dried blueberries instead.

Yellow Cake with Jam Topping

This was my mother's go-to cake when she had last-minute guests coming over. It's a dense, spongy cake with a sweet and tangy apricot or peach jam topping.

Yield:	Prep time:	Cook time:	Serving size:
1 (9×13-inch) cake; 16 pieces	20 minutes	20 minutes	1 piece

Each serving has:			
313 calories	8g fat	5g saturated fat	5g protein
57g carbohydrate	1g dietary fiber	84mg cholesterol	163mg sodium

5 large eggs

$1^1/_4$ cups sugar

1 TB. vanilla extract

2 cups all-purpose flour

2 tsp. baking powder

$^1/_2$ tsp. salt

$^1/_2$ cup whole milk

$^1/_2$ cup butter, melted

2 cups apricot or peach jam

$^1/_4$ cup sweetened condensed milk

2 TB. hot water

1. Preheat the oven to 350°F. Lightly coat a 9×13-inch cake pan with cooking spray, and dust with about 2 tablespoons all-purpose flour.

2. In a large bowl, and using an electric mixer on medium speed, beat eggs for 3 minutes.

3. Add sugar and vanilla extract, and beat for 2 more minutes.

4. Add all-purpose flour, baking powder, salt, whole milk, and melted butter, and blend for 1 minute.

5. Pour batter into the prepared pan, and bake for 20 minutes or until a toothpick inserted in center of cake comes out clean.

6. Cool cake completely.

7. In a small bowl, whisk together apricot jam, sweetened condensed milk, and hot water.

8. Pour jam icing over cake, letting it run over the edges, cut, and serve.

Mediterranean Doughnuts

These bite-size dough balls are flavored with traditional Mediterranean flavors and a touch of sweetness.

Yield:	Prep time:	Cook time:	Serving size:
3 dozen doughnuts	1¹/₂ hours	15 minutes	1 doughnut

Each serving has:			
138 calories	5g fat	4g saturated fat	1g protein
23g carbohydrate	1g dietary fiber	0mg cholesterol	1mg sodium

1 TB. active dry yeast	2 cups all-purpose flour
1 cup warm water	1 tsp. cinnamon
3 TB. sugar	8 cups vegetable oil
1 large potato, boiled, peeled, and mashed	4 cups Simple Syrup (recipe in Chapter 21)

1. In a large bowl, combine yeast, warm water, and sugar. Set aside for 5 minutes.

2. Add mashed potato, all-purpose flour, and cinnamon, and stir to combine. Cover with plastic wrap, and let sit for 1 hour.

3. In a large pot over medium heat, bring vegetable oil to 365°F.

4. Pour Simple Syrup in a large bowl.

5. Spoon up about 2 tablespoons dough mixture, drop into hot oil, and fry for 2 or 3 minutes or until dark brown.

6. Spoon out fried doughnuts from oil, and drop into Simple Syrup to soak for about 5 minutes.

7. Spoon out doughnuts from Simple Syrup, and place on a plate. Serve at room temperature.

 MEDITERRANEAN MORSEL

Potato might seem an odd ingredient to have in a dessert recipe! Here, it helps make the doughnuts a bit more dense and also acts as a binder.

Mediterranean Cheesecakes

This is a Mediterranean version of the traditional cheesecake recipe, with a toasted, shredded phyllo crust and a slightly sweet cream cheese filling.

Yield:	Prep time:	Cook time:	Serving size:
12 individual cheesecakes	2¼ hours	20 minutes	1 cheesecake

Each serving has:			
431 calories	23g fat	14g saturated fat	9g protein
48g carbohydrate	1g dietary fiber	82mg cholesterol	556mg sodium

4 cups shredded phyllo (kataifi dough)	1 TB. vanilla extract
½ cup butter, melted	2 TB. orange blossom water
12 oz. cream cheese	1 TB. orange zest
1 cup Greek yogurt	2 large eggs
¾ cup confectioners' sugar	1 cup coconut flakes

1. Preheat the oven to 450°F.

2. In a large bowl, and using your hands, combine shredded phyllo and melted butter, working the two together and breaking up phyllo shreds as you work.

3. Using a 12-cup muffin tin, add ⅓ cup shredded phyllo mixture to each tin, and press down to form crust on the bottom of the cup. Bake crusts for 8 minutes, remove from the oven, and set aside.

4. In a large bowl, and using an electric mixer on low speed, blend cream cheese and Greek yogurt for 1 minute.

5. Add confectioners' sugar, vanilla extract, orange blossom water, and orange zest, and blend 1 minute.

6. Add eggs, and blend for about 30 seconds or just until eggs are incorporated.

7. Lightly coat the sides of each muffin tin with cooking spray.

8. Pour about ⅓ cup cream cheese mixture over crust in each tin. Do not overflow.

9. Bake for 12 minutes.

10. Spread shredded coconut on a baking sheet, and place in the oven with cheesecakes to toast for 4 or 5 minutes or until golden brown. Remove from the oven, and set aside.

11. Remove cheesecakes from the oven, and cool for 1 hour on the countertop.

12. Place the tin in the refrigerator, and cool for 1 more hour.

13. To serve, dip a sharp knife in warm water and then run it along the sides of cheesecakes to loosen from the tin. Gently remove cheesecakes and place on a serving plate.

14. Sprinkle with toasted coconut flakes, and serve.

More Tempting Treats

In This Chapter

- Mouthwatering meal-enders
- Indulgent desserts
- Decadent drinks

In this chapter, you'll find indulgent desserts that will make your mouth water just thinking about them. Desserts can be part of a healthy diet, but it's very important to practice moderation when it comes to dessert. Don't make dessert an everyday affair. Instead, keep the focus on the day's other meals, and treat yourself to these special treats maybe once a week.

Coffee and tea are consumed daily in the Mediterranean culture. Coffee or tea is served at breakfast, lunch, dinner, and after dinner. Turkish or Greek coffee is the coffee of choice. It's a rich, bold coffee made with superfine coffee grounds. Recent studies have shown that Turkish coffee is actually beneficial to heart health because it helps facilitate the flow of blood to the heart. And studies show that tea is one of the best antioxidants you can consume. So the next time you're thinking about trying a new pick-me-up, try a cup of Turkish coffee or tea.

Halva (*Halawa*)

This sesame fudge is a very traditional dessert along the Mediterranean. Often, different types of nuts and chocolate are added to it for flavor.

Yield:	Prep time:	Cook time:	Serving size:
4 cups	10 minutes (2 days inactive)	10 minutes	$^1/_4$ cup

Each serving has:			
251 calories	15g fat	2g saturated fat	5g protein
30g carbohydrate	2g dietary fiber	0mg cholesterol	8mg sodium

$1^1/_2$ cups honey

$1^1/_2$ cups tahini paste

1 cup pistachios, coarsely chopped

1. Pour honey into a saucepan, set over low heat, and bring to 240°F.

2. In another saucepan over low heat, bring tahini paste to 120°F.

3. In a bowl, whisk together heated honey and tahini paste until smooth. Fold in pistachios.

4. Line a loaf pan with parchment paper and spray with cooking spray. Pour tahini mixture into the loaf pan, and refrigerate for 2 days to set.

5. Cut halva into bite-size pieces, and serve.

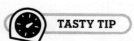 **TASTY TIP**

If you don't like pistachios, you can replace them with any other nut you like. Or for a more indulgent dessert, replace the pistachios with chocolate chips.

Custard Cookie Trifle

This trifle is made of slightly sweetened vanilla wafers, a yellow custard, and a bit of chocolate.

Yield:	Prep time:	Cook time:	Serving size:
1 (9×9-inch) trifle	20 minutes (2 hours inactive)	20 minutes	$^1/_{12}$ trifle

Each serving has:			
410 calories	20g fat	12g saturated fat	6g protein
50g carbohydrate	1g dietary fiber	113mg cholesterol	172mg sodium

1 cup sugar	3 TB. butter
$^1/_2$ cup all-purpose flour	1 TB. vanilla extract
$^1/_4$ tsp. salt	2 cups milk chocolate chips
3 cups whole milk	$^1/_2$ cup heavy cream
4 large egg yolks, beaten	40 vanilla wafers

1. In a large pot over medium heat, whisk together sugar, all-purpose flour, salt, and whole milk. Simmer for 4 minutes, continually stirring.

2. In a small bowl, whisk together egg yolks. While whisking, slowly pour 1 cup of hot milk mixture into eggs. Pour egg mixture back into the pot, continue to stir, and simmer for 2 minutes.

3. Stir in butter and vanilla extract until combined, and remove from heat.

4. Place milk chocolate chips and heavy cream in a bowl. Using a double boiler or a microwave, melt chocolate.

5. To form trifle, place a layer of vanilla wafers on the bottom of a 9×9-inch baking dish. Pour $^1/_2$ of custard mixture over cookies, drizzle $^1/_2$ of chocolate mixture over custard, and repeat, ending with a layer of chocolate on top.

6. Refrigerate for 2 hours before serving.

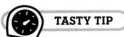 **TASTY TIP**

If you don't like or can't find vanilla wafers, you can use any plain cookie or cracker you like.

Rice Pudding

This creamy rice pudding is accented with hints of orange blossom and orange zest.

Yield:	Prep time:	Cook time:	Serving size:
6 cups	10 minutes	40 minutes	1 cup

Each serving has:			
412 calories	19g fat	12g saturated fat	6g protein
56g carbohydrate	1g dietary fiber	71mg cholesterol	81mg sodium

2 cups long-grain rice	2 TB. cornstarch
2$\frac{1}{2}$ cups water	1 tsp. orange zest
3$\frac{1}{2}$ cups whole milk	3 TB. orange blossom water
1 cup heavy cream	1 tsp. ground cinnamon
1 cup sugar	

1. In a large, 3-quart pot over medium heat, bring long-grain rice and 3 cups water to a simmer for 30 minutes.

2. Add whole milk, heavy cream, and sugar to rice, and simmer, stirring intermittently, for 20 minutes.

3. In a small bowl, dissolve cornstarch in remaining $\frac{1}{2}$ cup water. While stirring pudding, slowly pour in cornstarch mixture, add orange zest and orange blossom water, and simmer for 5 more minutes.

4. Pour pudding into a serving bowl or individual serving dishes, and cool at room temperature for 30 minutes.

5. Dust top of pudding with cinnamon, and serve at room temperature or refrigerate and serve cold.

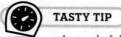 **TASTY TIP**

Instead of the orange zest and orange blossom water, you can substitute 1 vanilla bean. Scrape out the inside of the vanilla bean and add to the pudding when you add the cornstarch.

Mediterranean Bread Pudding (*Aish el Saraya*)

In this dessert, layered pieces of toasted bread are soaked in a flavored syrup and layered with a rich custard.

Yield:	Prep time:	Cook time:	Serving size:
1 (8×8-inch) pudding	20 minutes (4 hours inactive)	20 minutes	$^1/_9$ of pudding

Each serving has:			
437 calories	11g fat	5g saturated fat	6g protein
81g carbohydrate	2g dietary fiber	17mg cholesterol	251mg sodium

8 slices white bread, crust removed

1 cup sugar

$^1/_2$ cup water

1 TB. fresh lemon juice

2 cups Simple Syrup (recipe later in this chapter)

4 cups Ashta Custard (recipe later in this chapter)

$^1/_2$ cup coconut flakes, toasted

$^1/_2$ cup pistachios, ground

1 strawberry, sliced

1. Preheat the oven to 450°F.

2. Place slices of bread on a baking sheet, and toast for 10 minutes or until bread is golden brown and dry.

3. In a small saucepan over medium-low heat, combine sugar, water, and lemon juice. Simmer for 5 to 7 minutes or until sugar reaches a dark golden brown color.

4. Carefully pour hot dark brown syrup into an 8×8-inch baking dish, shifting the dish from side to side to spread syrup around bottom of dish.

5. Place 4 slices of bread on top of brown syrup. Pour 1 cup of Simple Syrup over bread, spread 2 cups Ashta Custard over bread, and add another layer of 4 slices of bread. Pour remaining 1 cup Simple Syrup over bread, and spread remaining 2 cups Ashta Custard over top bread layer.

6. Cover the dish with plastic wrap, and refrigerate for 4 hours.

7. Decorate top of dish with toasted coconut, pistachios, and strawberry slices, and serve.

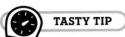 **TASTY TIP**

The longer you let this pudding sit, the better it is. Refrigerate it overnight before serving if you have the time.

Shredded Phyllo and Sweet Cheese Pie (*Knafe*)

This dessert combines crunchy shredded phyllo with a sweet cheese filling, all accented with a simple syrup.

Yield:	Prep time:	Cook time:	Serving size:
1 (9-inch-round) pie	20 minutes	30 minutes	$^1/_8$ pie

Each serving has:			
632 calories	37g fat	22g saturated fat	19g protein
56g carbohydrate	1g dietary fiber	96mg cholesterol	666mg sodium

1 lb. pkg. shredded phyllo (kataifi dough)

1 cup butter, melted

$^1/_2$ cup whole milk

2 TB. semolina flour

1 lb. ricotta cheese

2 cups mozzarella cheese, shredded

2 TB. sugar

1 cup Simple Syrup (recipe later in this chapter)

1. In a food processor fitted with a chopping blade, pulse shredded phyllo and butter 10 times. Transfer mixture to a bowl.

2. In a small saucepan over low heat, warm whole milk.

3. Stir in semolina flour, and cook for 1 minute.

4. Rinse the food processor, and to it, add ricotta cheese, mozzarella cheese, sugar, and semolina mixture. Blend for 1 minute.

5. Preheat the oven to 375°F.

6. In a 9-inch-round baking dish, add $^1/_2$ of shredded phyllo mixture, and press down to compress. Add cheese mixture, and spread out evenly. Add rest of shredded phyllo mixture, spread evenly, and gently press down. Bake for 40 minutes or until golden brown.

7. Let pie rest for 10 minutes before serving with Simple Syrup drizzled over top.

Fried Pancakes

These crunchy pancake pockets are filled with cheese, deep fried, and served with syrup.

Yield:	Prep time:	Cook time:	Serving size:
12 pancakes	45 minutes	30 minutes	1 pancake
Each serving has:			
331 calories	19g fat	14g saturated fat	6g protein
36g carbohydrate	1g dietary fiber	13mg cholesterol	175mg sodium

1 cup all-purpose flour	$^1/_2$ tsp. salt
$^1/_2$ cup whole-wheat flour	2 TB. sugar
1 cup whole milk	2 cups sweet cheese, shredded
$^1/_2$ cup water	8 cups vegetable oil
1 tsp. active dry yeast	1 cup Simple Syrup (recipe later in this chapter)
1 tsp. baking powder	

1. In a large bowl, whisk together all-purpose flour, whole-wheat flour, whole milk, water, yeast, baking powder, salt, and sugar. Set aside for 30 minutes.

2. Preheat a nonstick griddle over low heat.

3. Spoon 3 tablespoons batter onto the griddle, and cook pancake for about 30 seconds or until bubbles form along entire top of pancake. Do not flip over pancake. You're only browning the bottom.

4. Transfer pancake to a plate, and let cool while cooking remaining pancakes. Do not overlap pancakes while letting them cool.

5. Place 2 tablespoons sweet cheese in center of each pancake, fold over pancake, and tightly pinch it closed. Repeat with remaining pancakes.

6. In a large pot or fryer over medium heat, heat vegetable oil to 365°F.

7. Add 4 pancakes to hot oil, and fry for about 3 minutes or until dark brown. Remove fried pancake and place on a plate lined with paper towels. Repeat with remaining pancakes.

8. Drizzle fried pancake pockets with Simple Syrup, and serve warm or at room temperature.

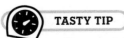 **TASTY TIP**

If you can't find sweet cheese, you can substitute fresh mozzarella instead. It melts just as well.

Custard-Filled Pancakes (*Atayef*)

These mini two-bite pancakes are filled with custard and make a fantastic dessert.

Yield:	Prep time:	Cook time:	Serving size:
12 pancakes	40 minutes	15 minutes	1 pancake

Each serving has:			
179 calories	4g fat	1g saturated fat	4g protein
32g carbohydrate	2g dietary fiber	6mg cholesterol	131mg sodium

1 cup all-purpose flour	2 TB. sugar
$^1/_2$ cup whole-wheat flour	2 cups Ashta Custard (recipe later in this chapter)
1 cup whole milk	$^1/_2$ cup ground pistachios
$^1/_2$ cup water	1 cup Simple Syrup (recipe later in this chapter)
1 tsp. active dry yeast	
1 tsp. baking powder	
$^1/_2$ tsp. salt	

1. In a large bowl, whisk together all-purpose flour, whole-wheat flour, whole milk, water, yeast, baking powder, salt, and sugar. Set aside for 30 minutes.

2. Preheat a nonstick griddle over low heat.

3. Spoon 3 tablespoons batter onto the griddle, and cook pancake for about 30 seconds or until bubbles form along entire top of pancake. Do not flip over pancake. You're only browning the bottom.

4. Transfer pancake to a plate, and let cool while cooking remaining pancakes. Do not overlap the pancakes while letting them cool.

5. Form pancake into a pocket by folding pancake into a half-moon, and pinch together the edges, but only halfway up.

6. Spoon Ashta Custard into a piping bag or a zipper-lock plastic bag, snip off the corner, and squeeze about 2 tablespoons custard into each pancake pocket. Sprinkle custard with pistachios.

7. Serve pancakes chilled with Simple Syrup drizzled on top.

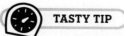 **TASTY TIP**

For best results, refrigerate the filled pancakes for 2 hours before serving. This firms them a bit.

Phyllo Custard Pockets (*Shaabiyat*)

These phyllo pockets are stuffed with a slightly sweetened custard and drizzled with a sweet simple syrup.

Yield:	Prep time:	Cook time:	Serving size:
12 pockets	15 minutes	10 minutes	1 pocket

Each serving has:			
225 calories	13g fat	7g saturated fat	3g protein
25g carbohydrate	1g dietary fiber	28mg cholesterol	152mg sodium

8 phyllo sheets

$^1/_2$ cup butter, melted

$2^1/_4$ cups Ashta Custard (recipe later in this chapter)

1 cup Simple Syrup (recipe later in this chapter)

$^1/_2$ cup pistachios, ground

1. Preheat the oven to 450°F.

2. Lay out a sheet of phyllo dough, brush with butter, and layer another sheet of phyllo dough on top. Cut sheets into 3 equal-size columns, each about 3 or 4 inches wide.

3. Place 3 tablespoons Ashta Custard at one end of each column, and fold the bottom-right corner up and over custard. Pull up bottom-left corner, and repeat folding each corner up to the opposite corner, forming a triangle as you fold.

4. Place triangle pockets on a baking sheet, brush with butter, and bake for 10 minutes or until golden brown.

5. Serve warm or cold, drizzled with Simple Syrup and sprinkled with pistachios.

Ashta Custard

This eggless custard, made with a smooth cream, makes for a really rich dessert.

Yield:	Prep time:	Cook time:	Serving size:
4 cups	10 minutes	9 minutes	2 tablespoons

Each serving has:			
32 calories	1g fat	1g saturated fat	1g protein
4g carbohydrate	0g dietary fiber	5mg cholesterol	24mg sodium

2 cups whole milk	3 TB. cornstarch
1 cup half-and-half	1/2 cup water
3 TB. sugar	2 TB. orange blossom water
5 pieces white bread, crust removed	2 TB. rose water

1. In a 2-quart pot over medium-low heat, combine whole milk, half-and-half, and sugar.

2. Cut white bread into small pieces, add to the pot, and whisk vigorously for about 1 minute. Continue whisking for about 5 minutes.

3. In a small bowl, dissolve cornstarch in water. Whisk cornstarch mixture into custard.

4. Stir orange blossom water and rose water into custard, and whisk for about 3 minutes. Custard should be very thick now.

5. Transfer custard to a bowl, and set on the countertop to cool for 1 hour.

6. Stir custard, cover with plastic wrap, and refrigerate for at least 3 hours before serving.

 TASTY TIP

This custard is great for any recipe that calls for a custard filling. You can swap out the orange blossom water and rose water with the flavoring of your choice to suit the recipe you want to use it for.

Sweet Cheese Rolls (*Halawet el Jibn*)

Sweet cheese is a combination of melted mozzarella cheese with semolina, forming a sweet cheese (hence the name) that's served with a creamy custard.

Yield:	Prep time:	Cook time:	Serving size:
12 rolls	25 minutes	5 minutes	1 roll
Each serving has:			
345 calories	15g fat	8.5g saturated fat	12g protein
40g carbohydrate	1g dietary fiber	40mg cholesterol	267mg sodium

$^1/_3$ cup butter

$^1/_2$ cup semolina

$^1/_2$ cup farina

$2^1/_2$ cups Simple Syrup (recipe later in this chapter)

1 lb. fresh mozzarella cheese, sliced

2 cups Ashta Custard (recipe earlier in this chapter)

2 TB. pistachios, ground

1. In a large pot over medium heat, cook butter, semolina, and farina for 3 minutes.

2. Add 1 cup Simple Syrup to the pot, stir, and cook for 3 minutes.

3. Add mozzarella to the pot, and cook, stirring vigorously, for about 3 minutes or until cheese is melted.

4. Pour $^1/_2$ cup Simple Syrup onto a baking sheet and spread out to coat all sides. Pour cheese mixture onto the baking sheet, and using the back of a wooden spoon, spread out to the size of the baking sheet. Cool for 15 minutes.

5. Run a knife down the baking sheet lengthwise, making two cuts in the sheet and forming three columns. Then make three more cuts widthwise, so you have 12 equal-size pieces.

6. Place 3 tablespoons Ashta Custard at one end of each piece, roll, place seam side down on a plate.

7. To serve, sprinkle each piece with ground pistachios and a drizzle of Simple Syrup.

Mascarpone-Stuffed Dates

I love this dessert because it's bite sized and there's no baking involved. The natural sweetness of the dates with the creamy flavor of the mascarpone makes this an indulgent dessert.

Yield:	Prep time:	Cook time:	Serving size:
12 dates	40 minutes	5 minutes	1 date

Each serving has:			
168 calories	10g fat	4g saturated fat	2g protein
20g carbohydrate	2g dietary fiber	18mg cholesterol	13mg sodium

12 medjool dates

$^1/_2$ cup pecans, ground

$^1/_4$ cup coconut flakes

6 oz. mascarpone cheese

1. Preheat the oven to 450°F.

2. Slice medjool dates lengthwise, remove pits, and slightly open dates.

3. Spread ground pecans in an even layer on a baking sheet. Spread coconut flakes evenly on another baking sheet. Toast pecans for 3 minutes. Toast coconut for 5 minutes.

4. In a small bowl, combine $^1/_2$ of toasted ground pecans and all of toasted coconuts. Add the mascarpone cheese and stir to combine. Place mixture in a piping bag or a zipper-lock plastic bag, and cut off corner of bag.

5. Place remaining pecans in a bowl.

6. Pipe out about 1 tablespoon cheese mixture into each date, and slightly close dates around filling. Dip exposed cheese part of dates into toasted pecans, and set stuffed dates on a serving platter.

7. Refrigerate for 30 minutes before serving.

 MEDITERRANEAN MORSEL

You can make these up to 2 days in advance and store them covered in the refrigerator until you're ready to serve.

Mediterranean Fruit Tart

This light and flavorful fruit tart combines a sweet custard with fresh fruit and a flaky crust.

Yield:	Prep time:	Cook time:	Serving size:
1 (9-inch) tart	40 minutes	15 minutes	$^1/_8$ of tart
Each serving has:			
644 calories	39g fat	20g saturated fat	6g protein
70g carbohydrate	2g dietary fiber	71mg cholesterol	375mg sodium

$2^1/_4$ cups all-purpose flour

$^1/_2$ tsp. salt

2 TB. sugar

1 cup cold butter

$^1/_2$ cup shortening

5 TB. ice water

2 cups Ashta Custard (recipe earlier in this chapter)

10 strawberries, sliced

2 kiwi, peeled and sliced

1 cup blueberries

1 cup peach or apricot jam

3 TB. water

1. In a food processor fitted with a chopping blade, pulse 2 cups all-purpose flour, salt, and sugar 5 times.

2. Add butter and shortening, and blend for 1 minute or until mixture is crumbly. Transfer mixture to a medium bowl.

3. Add ice water to batter, and mix just until combined.

4. Place dough on a piece of plastic wrap, form into a flat disc, and refrigerate for 20 minutes.

5. Preheat the oven to 450°F.

6. Dust your workspace with flour, and using a rolling pin, roll out dough to $^1/_8$ inch thickness. Place rolled-out dough into a 9-inch tart pan, press to mold into pan, and cut off excess dough. Bake for 13 minutes.

7. Let tart cool for 10 minutes.

8. Place tart shell on a serving dish, and fill with Ashta Custard. Arrange strawberry slices, kiwi slices, and blueberries on top of tart.

9. In a small saucepan over medium heat, heat peach jam and water, stirring, for 2 minutes.

10. Using a pastry brush, brush top of fruit and tart with warmed jam.

11. Serve chilled and store in the refrigerator.

Fruit Salad

This is not your typical fruit salad. It combines fresh fruit with a sweet and tangy dressing.

Yield:	Prep time:	Serving size:	
12 cups	15 minutes	1 cup	

Each serving has:			
100 calories	0g fat	0g saturated fat	1g protein
25g carbohydrate	3g dietary fiber	0mg cholesterol	2mg sodium

10 large strawberries, diced	1 large mango, peeled and diced
3 large kiwi, peeled and diced	2 large bananas, sliced
1 cup blueberries	1 cup fresh orange juice
1 large peach, diced	3 TB. honey
1 large pear, peeled and diced	2 TB. orange blossom water
1 large grapefruit, peeled and sectioned	2 TB. rose water

1. In a large bowl, combine strawberries, kiwi, blueberries, peach, pear, grapefruit, mango, and bananas.

2. In a small bowl, whisk together orange juice, honey, orange blossom water, and rose water.

3. Pour dressing over fruit, and gently toss.

4. Keep salad refrigerated, and serve cold.

 MEDITERRANEAN MORSEL

Feel free to use whatever fruit is in season for this recipe. Usually when fruit is in season, its flavor is brighter and sweeter.

Simple Syrup

This simple syrup has wonderful undertones of orange blossoms and rose petals. It's easy to make and great for using as a dessert topping.

Yield:	Prep time:	Cook time:	Serving size:
3 cups	5 minutes	15 minutes	2 tablespoons

Each serving has:			
65 calories	0g fat	0g saturated fat	0g protein
17g carbohydrate	0g dietary fiber	0mg cholesterol	0mg sodium

2 cups sugar

1 cup water

2 TB. fresh lemon juice

2 TB. orange blossom water

2 TB. rose water

1. In a medium saucepan over low heat, combine sugar, water, and lemon juice. Simmer for 14 minutes or until syrup starts to thicken and coats the back of a spoon.

2. Stir in orange blossom water and rose water, and simmer for 1 more minute. Remove from heat, and let cool to room temperature.

3. Store in a glass jar in the refrigerator for up to 1 month.

 MEDITERRANEAN MORSEL

This syrup is even great served over pancakes or waffles!

Turkish Coffee (Greek Coffee)

This coffee is very strong but is actually very healthy for your heart. It has a bold flavor but is smooth on your palate.

Yield:	Prep time:	Cook time:	Serving size:
1 cup	2 minutes	3 minutes	$^1/_3$ cup

Each serving has:			
17 calories	0g fat	0g saturated fat	0g protein
4g carbohydrate	0g dietary fiber	0mg cholesterol	1mg sodium

1 cup water   4 TB. ground Turkish coffee

1 TB. sugar

1. In a small pot or Turkish coffee pot over low heat, combine water, sugar, and Turkish coffee. Simmer, stirring, for 3 minutes, allowing foam to form on top of coffee. Be careful not to let coffee to boil over. If coffee seems to rise, remove from heat for 5 seconds and then return to heat and continue cooking.

2. Let coffee sit for 3 minutes, allowing coffee grounds to settle to the bottom of the pot.

3. Serve warm in an espresso cup with some foam on top.

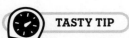 **TASTY TIP**

Some people like to add ground cardamom to Turkish coffee. If you like that flavor, add $^1/_8$ teaspoon ground cardamom to the coffee pot when you add the ground coffee.

Cinnamon Tea

This tea is served at special events in the Mediterranean region. It has a very subtle, soothing cinnamon flavor, with light notes of tea.

Yield:	Prep time:	Cook time:	Serving size:
6 cups	10 minutes	32 minutes	1 cup

Each serving has:			
28 calories	0g fat	0g saturated fat	0g protein
7g carbohydrate	1g dietary fiber	0mg cholesterol	1mg sodium

6 cups water

1 (3-in.) cinnamon stick

6 TB. Ahmad Tea, Ceylon tea, or
   your favorite

3 TB. sugar

1. In a teapot over low heat, bring water and cinnamon stick to a simmer for 30 minutes. Remove cinnamon stick.

2. Stir in Ahmad tea and sugar, and simmer for 2 minutes.

3. Remove from heat, and let sit for 10 minutes.

4. Strain tea into tea cups, and serve warm.

Glossary

al dente   Italian for "against the teeth," this term refers to pasta or rice that's neither soft nor hard but just slightly firm against the teeth.

all-purpose flour   Flour that contains only the inner part of the wheat grain. It's suitable for everything from cakes to gravies.

allspice   A spice named for its flavor echoes of several spices (cinnamon, cloves, nutmeg) used in many desserts and in rich marinades and stews.

amino acid   An organic chemical compound that makes up proteins.

antioxidant   A substance that protects your cells from the damage caused by free radicals.

arborio rice   A plump Italian rice used for, among other purposes, risotto.

artichoke heart   The center part of the artichoke flower, often found canned in grocery stores.

arugula   A spicy-peppery green with leaves that resemble a dandelion and have a distinctive and very sharp flavor.

bake   To cook in a dry oven. Dry-heat cooking often results in a crisping of the exterior of the food being cooked. Moist-heat cooking, through methods such as steaming, poaching, etc., brings a much different, moist quality to the food.

baking powder   A dry ingredient used to increase volume and lighten or leaven baked goods.

balsamic vinegar   Vinegar produced primarily in Italy from a specific type of grape and aged in wood barrels. It's heavier, darker, and sweeter than most vinegars.

barley   A cereal grain with a nutty flavor that's high in protein and fiber.

basil   A flavorful, almost sweet, resinous herb delicious with tomatoes and used in all kinds of Italian- or Mediterranean-style dishes.

baste   To keep foods moist during cooking by spooning, brushing, or drizzling with a liquid.

beat   To quickly mix substances.

Belgian endive   *See* endive.

blanch   To place a food in boiling water for about 1 minute or less to partially cook the exterior and then submerge in or rinse with cool water to halt the cooking.

blend   To completely mix something, usually with a blender or food processor, slower than beating.

boil   To heat a liquid to the point where water is forced to turn into steam, causing the liquid to bubble. To boil something is to insert it into boiling water. A rapid boil is when a lot of bubbles form on the surface of the liquid.

bok choy   A member of the cabbage family with thick stems, crisp texture, and fresh flavor. It's perfect for stir-frying.

braise   To cook with the introduction of some liquid, usually over an extended period of time.

brine   A highly salted, often seasoned, liquid used to flavor and preserve foods. To brine a food is to soak, or preserve, it by submerging it in brine. The salt in the brine penetrates the fibers of the meat and makes it moist and tender.

broil   To cook in a dry oven under the overhead high-heat element.

broth   *See* stock.

brown   To cook in a skillet, turning, until the food's surface is seared and brown in color, to lock in the juices.

brown rice   A whole-grain rice, including the germ, with a characteristic pale brown or tan color. It's more nutritious and flavorful than white rice.

bulgur   A wheat kernel that's been steamed, dried, and crushed and is sold in fine and coarse textures.

cake flour   A high-starch, soft, and fine flour used primarily for cakes.

caper   The flavorful buds of a Mediterranean plant, ranging in size from *nonpareil* (about the size of a small pea) to larger, grape-size caper berries produced in Spain.

caramelize   To cook sugar over low heat until it develops a sweet caramel flavor, or to cook vegetables (especially onions) or meat in butter or oil over low heat until they soften, sweeten, and develop a caramel color.

caraway   A distinctive spicy seed used for bread, pork, cheese, and cabbage dishes. It's known to reduce stomach upset, which is why it's often paired with foods like sauerkraut.

carbohydrate   A main nutrient and important source of energy for your body to function.

cardamom   An intense, sweet-smelling spice used in baking and coffee and common in Indian cooking.

cardiovascular disease   A disease that involves blood vessels, the heart, or both. It affects the cardiovascular system, which includes veins, arteries, and capillaries.

carob   A tropical tree that produces long pods from which the dried, baked, and powdered flesh—carob powder—is used in baking. The flavor is sweet and reminiscent of chocolate.

carotenoid   A plant pigment that gives color to tomatoes and leaves. Your body converts it to vitamin A, a strong antioxidant.

cayenne   A fiery spice made from hot chile peppers, especially the cayenne chile, a slender, red, and very hot pepper.

ceviche   A seafood dish in which fresh fish or seafood is marinated for several hours in highly acidic lemon or lime juice, tomato, onion, and cilantro. The acid "cooks" the seafood.

chevre   A creamy-salty soft goat cheese. Chevres vary in style from mild and creamy to aged, firm, and flavorful.

chickpea (or **garbanzo bean**)   A yellow-gold, roundish bean used as the base ingredient in hummus. Chickpeas are high in fiber and low in fat.

chile (or **chili**)   Any one of many different "hot" peppers, ranging in intensity from the relatively mild ancho pepper to the blisteringly hot habañero.

chili powder   A warm, rich seasoning blend that includes chile pepper, cumin, garlic, and oregano.

Chinese five-spice powder   A pungent mixture of equal parts cinnamon, cloves, fennel seed, anise, and Szechuan peppercorns.

chive   A member of the onion family, chives grow in bunches of long leaves that resemble tall grass or the green tops of onions and offer a light onion flavor.

cholesterol   A fat produced by the liver that's found in every cell in the human body. It's essential for body function, but it can be detrimental if present in high levels.

chop   To cut into pieces, usually qualified by an adverb such as "*coarsely* chopped" or by a size measurement such as "chopped into $1/2$-inch pieces." "Finely chopped" is much closer to mince.

chorizo   A spiced pork sausage that can be eaten alone or as a component in many recipes, usually Mexican.

chutney   A thick condiment often served with Indian curries made with fruits and/or vegetables with vinegar, sugar, and spices.

cider vinegar   A vinegar produced from apple cider, popular in North America.

cilantro   A member of the parsley family used in Mexican dishes (especially salsa) and some Asian dishes. Use in moderation because the flavor can overwhelm. The seed of the cilantro plant is the spice coriander.

cinnamon   A rich, aromatic spice commonly used in baking or desserts. Cinnamon can also be used for delicious and interesting entrées.

clove   A sweet, strong, almost wintergreen-flavor spice used in baking.

complex carbohydrate   A nutrient made of three sugar molecules instead of two. Complex carbs help your body convert glucose to energy. It takes longer for your body to break them down, therefore, helping regulate blood sugar levels.

coriander   A rich, warm, spicy seed used in all types of recipes, from African to South American, from entrées to desserts.

cornstarch   A thickener used in baking and food processing. It's the refined starch of the endosperm of the corn kernel and often mixed with cold liquid to make into a paste before adding to a recipe to avoid clumps.

coronary heart disease   The buildup of plaque in the arteries of the heart.

couscous   Granular semolina (durum wheat) that's cooked and used in many Mediterranean and North African dishes.

cream   To beat a fat such as butter, often with another ingredient such as sugar, to soften and aerate a batter.

crimini mushroom   A relative of the white button mushroom that's brown in color and has a richer flavor. The larger, fully grown version is the portobello. *See also* portobello mushroom.

crudité   Fresh vegetables served as an appetizer, often all together on one tray.

cumin   A fiery, smoky-tasting spice popular in Middle Eastern and Indian dishes. Cumin is a seed; ground cumin seed is the most common form used in cooking.

curry   Rich, spicy, Indian-style sauces and the dishes prepared with them. A curry uses curry powder as its base seasoning.

curry powder   A ground blend of rich and flavorful spices used as a basis for curry and many other Indian-influenced dishes. Common ingredients include hot pepper, nutmeg, cumin, cinnamon, pepper, and turmeric. Some curry can also be found in paste form.

custard   A cooked mixture of eggs and milk popular as a base for desserts.

dash   A few drops, usually of a liquid, released by a quick shake.

deglaze   To scrape up bits of meat and seasoning left in a pan or skillet after cooking. Usually this is done by adding a liquid such as wine or broth and creating a flavorful stock that can be used to create sauces.

devein   To remove the dark vein from the back of a large shrimp with a sharp knife.

diabetes   A disease in which the body has no ability to produce insulin, which causes high levels of glucose to remain in the blood.

dice   To cut into small cubes about $1/4$-inch square.

Dijon mustard   A hearty, spicy mustard made in the style of the Dijon region of France.

dill   A herb perfect for eggs, salmon, cheese dishes, and, of course, vegetables (pickles!).

docosahexaenoic acid (DHA)   A fatty acid found in cold-water fish that improves brain function, helps thin blood, and lowers triglyceride levels. It also helps prevent type 2 diabetes, coronary artery disease, dementia, and attention deficit hyperactivity disorder (ADHD).

double boiler   A set of two pots designed to nest together, one inside the other, and provide consistent, moist heat for foods that need delicate treatment. The bottom pot holds water (not quite touching the bottom of the top pot); the top pot holds the food you want to heat.

dredge   To coat a piece of food on all sides with a dry substance such as flour or cornmeal.

drizzle   To lightly sprinkle drops of a liquid over food, often as the finishing touch to a dish.

edamame   Fresh, plump, pale green soybeans, similar in appearance to lima beans, often served steamed and either shelled or still in their protective pods.

eicosapentaenoic acid (EPA)   A fatty acid found in cold-water fish that prevents blood from clotting and helps reduce pain and swelling. It's used to regulate high blood pressure, heart disease, Alzheimer's disease, personality disorders, depression, and diabetes.

endive   A green that resembles a small, elongated, tightly packed head of romaine lettuce. The thick, crunchy leaves can be broken off and used with dips and spreads.

entrée   The main dish in a meal.

extra-virgin olive oil   *See* olive oil.

extract   A concentrated flavoring derived from foods or plants through evaporation or distillation that imparts a powerful flavor without altering the volume or texture of a dish.

falafel   A Middle Eastern food made of seasoned, ground chickpeas formed into balls, cooked, and often used as a filling in pitas.

farina   A cereal grain often referred to as cream of wheat. It's usually served warm as a breakfast food but has many other uses in baking or pasta-making.

fennel   In seed form, a fragrant, licorice-tasting herb. The bulbs have a mild flavor and a celery-like crunch and are used as a vegetable in salads or cooked recipes.

flour   Grains ground into a meal. Wheat is perhaps the most common flour, but oats, rye, buckwheat, soybeans, chickpeas, etc. can also be used. *See also* all-purpose flour; cake flour; whole-wheat flour.

fold   To combine a dense and light mixture with a circular action from the middle of the bowl.

free radical   An electron that has broken its bond with another electron and attacks another molecule in order to attach to its electron, setting up a chain reaction in the body.

freekeh   A green wheat that's roasted and has a smoky, earthy flavor.

frittata   A skillet-cooked mixture of eggs and other ingredients that's not stirred but is cooked slowly and then either flipped or finished under the broiler.

fructose   Fruit sugar, a simple monosaccharide, found in plants.

fry   *See* sauté.

garlic   A member of the onion family, a pungent and flavorful vegetable used in many savory dishes. A garlic bulb contains multiple cloves. Each clove, when chopped, provides about 1 teaspoon garlic.

ginger   A flavorful root available fresh or dried and ground that adds a pungent, sweet, and spicy quality to a dish.

glucose   A simple sugar found in plants.

Greek yogurt   A strained yogurt that's a good natural source of protein, calcium, and probiotics. Greek yogurt averages 40 percent more protein per ounce than traditional yogurt.

halloumi cheese   An unripened brined cheese that originated in Cyprus and is very popular in Greece, Turkey, and Lebanon. It has a high melting point, so it's great for frying or grilling.

handful   An unscientific measurement, it's the amount of an ingredient you can hold in your hand.

healthy fat   Fat that's unsaturated. Healthy fats include omega-3 fatty acids, monounsaturated fats, and polyunsaturated fats. These good fats can lower cholesterol and reduce the risk of heart disease.

hearts of palm   Firm, elongated, off-white cylinders from the inside of a palm tree stem tip.

heme iron   Iron found in foods that contain hemoglobin, such as red meat, poultry, and fish.

herbes de Provence   A seasoning mix of basil, fennel, marjoram, rosemary, sage, and thyme, common in the south of France.

hoisin sauce   A sweet Asian condiment similar to ketchup made with soybeans, sesame, chile peppers, and sugar.

horseradish   A sharp, spicy root that forms the flavor base in condiments such as cocktail sauce and sharp mustards. Prepared horseradish contains vinegar and oil, among other ingredients. Use pure horseradish much more sparingly than the prepared version, or try cutting it with sour cream.

hummus   A thick, Middle Eastern spread made of puréed chickpeas, lemon juice, olive oil, garlic, and often tahini.

hydrogenation   The process of adding hydrogen to a product, including oils and fats like shortening, to extend its shelf life.

hypertension   High blood pressure, or when the arteries have a higher pressure of blood pushing through them.

infusion   A liquid in which flavorful ingredients such as herbs have been soaked or steeped to extract their flavor into the liquid.

Italian seasoning   A blend of dried herbs, including basil, oregano, rosemary, and thyme.

Jew's mallow leaf   The leaf of the jute plant. It's used to make stew.

jicama   A juicy, crunchy, sweet, large, round Central American vegetable. If you can't find jicama, try substituting sliced water chestnuts.

julienne   A French word meaning "to slice into very thin pieces."

kalamata olive   Traditionally from Greece, a medium-small, long black olive with a rich, smoky flavor.

Key lime   A very small lime grown primarily in Florida known for its tart taste.

knead   To work dough to make it pliable so it holds gas bubbles as it bakes. Kneading is fundamental in the process of making yeast breads.

kosher salt   A coarse-grained salt made without any additives or iodine.

lactose   The sugar found in milk products.

legume   A plant that has a dried "fruit" that's held inside a pod. Common legumes include green beans, peas, lentils, alfalfa, peanuts, and most other beans.

lentil   A tiny lens-shape pulse used in European, Middle Eastern, and Indian cuisines.

marinate   To soak meat, seafood, or another food in a seasoned sauce, a marinade, that's high in acid content. The acids break down the muscle of the meat, making it tender and adding flavor.

marjoram   A sweet herb, cousin of and similar to oregano popular in Greek, Spanish, and Italian dishes.

Mediterranean diet pyramid   A nutritional guide developed by Oldways, Harvard school of Public Health, and The World Health Organization in 1993.

meld   To allow flavors to blend and spread over time. Melding is often why recipes call for overnight refrigeration and is also why some dishes taste better as leftovers.

meringue   A baked mixture of sugar and beaten egg whites, often used as a dessert topping.

mesclun   Mixed salad greens, usually containing lettuce and other assorted greens such as arugula, cress, and endive.

metabolism   The life-sustaining chemical transformations of cells inside your body.

millet   A tiny, round, yellow-colored nutty-flavored grain often used as a replacement for couscous.

mince   To cut into very small pieces, smaller than diced, about $1/8$ inch or smaller.

mineral   A naturally occurring element from the earth that helps your body grow. Minerals are usually found in the earth but are also found in traces in fruits, vegetables, and meats.

miso   A fermented, flavorful soybean paste, key in many Japanese dishes.

nonheme iron   Iron found in nonanimal foods like vegetables and grains.

nutmeg   A sweet, fragrant, musky spice used primarily in baking.

olive   The fruit of the olive tree commonly grown on all sides of the Mediterranean. Black olives are also called ripe olives. Green olives are immature, although they're also widely eaten. *See also* kalamata olives.

olive oil   A fragrant liquid produced by crushing or pressing olives. Extra-virgin olive oil—the most flavorful and highest quality—is produced from the first pressing of a batch of olives; oil is also produced from later pressings.

omega-3 fatty acid   An unsaturated heart-healthy fat that's usually found in fish oils. It helps protect against many chronic diseases.

oregano   A fragrant, slightly astringent herb used in Greek, Spanish, and Italian dishes.

orzo   A rice-shape pasta used in Greek cooking.

oxidation   The browning of fruit flesh that happens over time and with exposure to air. Minimize oxidation by rubbing the cut surfaces with lemon juice.

paella   A Spanish dish of rice, shellfish, onion, meats, rich broth, and herbs.

paprika   A rich, red, warm, earthy spice that lends a rich red color to many dishes.

parboil   To partially cook in boiling water or broth.

parsley   A fresh-tasting green leafy herb, often used as a garnish.

pesto   A thick spread or sauce made with fresh basil leaves, garlic, olive oil, pine nuts, and Parmesan cheese.

phyllo dough   A pastry dough made of very thin sheets of dough. Usually each layer is brushed with butter to create a flaky crust.

pilaf   A rice dish in which the rice is browned in butter or oil and then cooked in a flavorful liquid such as a broth, often with the addition of meats or vegetables.

pinch   An unscientific measurement for the amount of an ingredient—typically, a dry, granular substance such as an herb or seasoning—you can hold between your finger and thumb.

pine nut   A nut that's rich (high in fat), flavorful, and a bit pine-y. Pine nuts are a traditional ingredient in pesto and add a hearty crunch to many other recipes.

pita bread   A flat, hollow wheat bread often used for sandwiches or sliced pizza style. They're terrific soft with dips or baked or broiled as a vehicle for other ingredients.

pizza stone   A flat stone that when preheated with the oven, cooks crusts to a crispy, pizza-parlor texture.

poach   To cook a food in simmering liquid such as water, wine, or broth.

polenta   A mush made from cornmeal that can be eaten hot with butter or cooked until firm and cut into squares.

porcini mushroom   A rich and flavorful mushroom used in rice and Italian-style dishes.

portobello mushroom   A mature and larger form of the smaller crimini mushroom. Brown, chewy, and flavorful, portobellos are often served as whole caps, grilled, or as thin sautéed slices. *See also* crimini mushrooms.

preheat   To turn on an oven, broiler, or other cooking appliance in advance of cooking so the temperature will be at the desired level when the assembled dish is ready for cooking.

probiotics   Microorganisms that offer health benefits to your body, especially your digestive and immune systems.

prosciutto   A dry, salt-cured ham that originated in Italy.

protein   A large, complex molecule made up of amino acids that plays an important role in many of your body's functions.

purée   To reduce a food to a thick, creamy texture, typically using a blender or food processor.

quinoa   A nutty-flavored seed that's extremely high in protein and calcium.

reduce   To boil or simmer a broth or sauce to remove some of the water content, resulting in more concentrated flavor and color.

refined grain   A grain that's significantly modified and has the bran and germ removed.

render   To cook a meat to the point where its fat melts and can be removed.

rice vinegar   Vinegar produced from fermented rice or rice wine, popular in Asian-style dishes. (It's not the same thing as rice wine vinegar.)

risotto   A popular Italian rice dish made by browning arborio rice in butter or oil and then slowly adding liquid to cook the rice, resulting in a creamy texture.

roast   To cook something uncovered in an oven, usually without additional liquid.

rosemary   A pungent, sweet herb used with chicken, pork, fish, and especially lamb. A little goes a long way.

roux   A mixture of butter or another fat and flour used to thicken sauces and soups.

saffron   An expensive spice made from the stamens of crocus flowers. Saffron lends a dramatic yellow color and distinctive flavor to a dish. Use only tiny amounts.

sage   An herb with a musty yet fruity, lemon-rind scent and "sunny" flavor.

saturated fat   A fat that's made of triglycerides containing only saturated fatty acids and carbon atoms completely saturated with hydrogen atoms. It's usually solid at room temperature and comes from mainly animal sources.

sauté   To pan-cook over lower heat than what's used for frying.

savory   A popular herb with a fresh, woody taste. Can also describe the flavor of food.

scald   To heat milk just until it's about to boil and then remove it from heat. Scalding milk helps prevent it from souring.

scant   An ingredient measurement directive not to add any extra, perhaps even leaving the measurement a tad short.

sear   To quickly brown the exterior of a food, especially meat, over high heat.

semolina   A by-product of milling wheat, like durum wheat. It's used in many products such as couscous, pasta, and cereals. It's also used in many baked goods.

sesame oil   An oil made from pressing sesame seeds. It's tasteless if clear and aromatic and flavorful if brown.

seven spice mix   A Mediterranean spice mix commonly used to season dishes.

shallot   A member of the onion family that grows in a bulb somewhat like garlic but has a milder onion flavor. When a recipe calls for shallot, use the entire bulb.

shellfish A broad range of seafood, including clams, mussels, oysters, crabs, shrimp, and lobster.

shiitake mushroom A large, dark brown mushroom with a hearty, meaty flavor. It can be used fresh or dried, grilled, as a component in other recipes, and as a flavoring source for broth.

short-grain rice A starchy rice popular in Asian-style dishes because it readily clumps, making it perfect for eating with chopsticks.

simmer To boil gently so the liquid barely bubbles.

simple carbohydrate A simple sugar composed of only one or two sugars; refined sugar. It has little to no nutritional value.

skim To remove fat or other material from the top of liquid.

smoke point The temperature at which an oil begins to break down or burn.

steam To suspend a food over boiling water and allow the heat of the steam (water vapor) to cook the food. This quick-cooking method preserves a food's flavor and texture.

steep To let sit in hot water, as in steeping tea in hot water for 10 minutes.

stew To slowly cook pieces of food submerged in a liquid. Also, a dish prepared by this method.

sticky rice *See* short-grain rice.

stir-fry To cook small pieces of food in a wok or skillet over high heat, moving and turning the food quickly to cook all sides.

stock A flavorful broth made by cooking meats and/or vegetables with seasonings until the liquid absorbs these flavors. The liquid is strained and the solids are discarded.

strata A savory bread pudding made with eggs and cheese.

sumac A fruit of a flowering plant that's dried and ground and has a tart, tangy flavor.

tahini A paste made from sesame seeds used to flavor many Middle Eastern recipes.

tamarind A sweet, pungent, flavorful fruit used in Indian-style sauces and curries.

tapenade A thick, chunky spread made from savory ingredients such as olives, lemon juice, and anchovies.

tarragon A sweet, rich-smelling herb perfect with seafood, vegetables (especially asparagus), chicken, and pork.

tempeh An Indonesian food made by culturing and fermenting soybeans into a cake, sometimes mixed with grains or vegetables. It's high in protein and fiber.

teriyaki A Japanese-style sauce composed of soy sauce, rice wine, ginger, and sugar that works well with seafood as well as most meats.

thyme   A minty, zesty herb.

tofu   A cheeselike substance made from soybeans and soy milk.

turmeric   A spicy, pungent yellow root used in many dishes, especially Indian cuisine, for color and flavor. Turmeric is the source of the yellow color in many prepared mustards.

type 2 diabetes   A disease in which the body can produce insulin but not in levels effective for the body to break down glucose, leaving glucose in the blood and damaging the body's tissues.

tzatziki   A Greek dip traditionally made with Greek yogurt, cucumbers, garlic, and mint.

vinegar   An acidic liquid widely used as a dressing and seasoning, often made from fermented grapes, apples, or rice. *See also* balsamic vinegar; cider vinegar; rice vinegar; white vinegar; wine vinegar.

vitamin   An organic compound required by the body to sustain life.

water chestnut   A tuber popular in many Asian dishes. It's white, crunchy, and juicy, and holds its texture whether cool or hot.

whisk   To rapidly mix, introducing air to the mixture.

white mushroom   A button mushroom. When fresh, white mushrooms have an earthy smell and an appealing soft crunch.

white vinegar   The most common type of vinegar, produced from grain.

whole grain   A grain derived from the seeds of grasses, including rice, oats, rye, wheat, wild rice, quinoa, barley, buckwheat, bulgur, corn, millet, amaranth, and sorghum.

whole-wheat flour   Wheat flour that contains the entire grain.

wild rice   Not a rice at all, this is actually a grass. It has a rich, nutty flavor and serves as a nutritious side dish.

wine vinegar   Vinegar produced from red or white wine.

yeast   Tiny fungi that, when mixed with water, sugar, flour, and heat, release carbon dioxide bubbles, which, in turn, cause the bread to rise.

zaatar   A Middle Eastern herb spice mix used as a versatile seasoning.

zest   Small slivers of peel, usually from a citrus fruit such as a lemon, lime, or orange.

Index

A

Aish el Saraya (Mediterranean Bread Pudding), 253
appetizers
    Aromatic Artichokes, 143
    Beef Tartar , 147
    Cheese Rolls, 144
    Hummus Appetizer Bites, 142
    Meat-Filled Phyllo, 146
    Savory Pita Chips, 149
    Spinach Pies, 145
Aromatic Artichokes, 143
artichokes, Aromatic Artichokes, 143
Ashta Custard, 258
Atayef (Custard-Filled Pancakes), 256

B

Baba Ganoush, 140
Baked Salmon, 202
Baked Spaghetti with Beef, 88-89
Baklava, 233-234
Bamya (Okra Stew), 81
Barley and Chicken Soup, 76
Basil and Shrimp Quinoa, 102
Batata Harra (Spicy Herb Potatoes), 217
Bazella (Green Pea Stew), 82
beans
    Bean Salad, 62
    Breakfast Beans (Ful Mudammas), 43
    Green Bean Stew, 84

    Green Fava Beans, 218
    Lentils and Bulgur Wheat Pilaf, 126
    Lentils and Rice, 125
    White Bean Hummus, 134
beef recipes
    Baked Spaghetti with Beef, 88-89
    Beef and Vegetable Soup, 68
    Beef-Stuffed Baked Potatoes, 91
    Beef-Stuffed Squash (Kusa Mihshi), 90
    Beef Tartar, 147
    Beefy Pita Sandwiches, 86
    Cheeseless Meat Pizza (Lahme bi Ajeen), 94
    Hearty Meat and Potatoes, 89
    Hummus with Meat, 131
    Kefta Burgers, 87
    main dishes
        Beef and Potatoes with Tahini Sauce, 178-179
        Beef Shawarma, 166
        Beef Shish Kabobs, 170-171
        Dumplings in Yogurt Sauce, 176-177
        Kefta Kabob, 167
        Kibbeh in a Pan, 169-170
        Kibbeh with Yogurt, 168-169
        Meat and Rice-Stuffed Grape Leaves, 174
        Square Meat Pies, 175
        Stuffed Eggplant Casserole, 179-180
        Stuffed Squash Casserole, 177-178

        Tomato and Beef Casserole, 171-172
    Meat-Filled Phyllo, 146
    Spiced Meat and Rice, 222
beets, Roasted Beet Salad, 55-56
benefits (health benefits)
    disease prevention, 4-5
    nutritional, 6
    weight loss, 5-6
Braised Chicken, 194
Braised Lamb and Tomatoes, 183
Breaded Chicken (Chicken Escalope), 95-96
breads
    Multipurpose Dough, 151
    Pita Bread, 148-149
    Rosemary Olive Bread, 150
    Sweet Bread with Dates, 45-46
Breakfast Beans (*Ful Mudammas*), 43
Breakfast Casserole (*Fatteh*), 38-39
breakfast recipes, 27
    Breakfast Beans (*Ful Mudammas*), 43
    Breakfast Casserole (*Fatteh*), 38-39
    Cheesy Breakfast Pizza (Cheese *Manakish*), 41-42
    Fried Cheese, 36
    Garlic Scrambled Eggs, 31
    Herbed Potatoes and Eggs, 35
    Holiday Eggs, 32
    Mediterranean Breakfast Quiche, 39-40
    Mediterranean Omelet, 33
    Potatoes and Eggs Omelet, 34
    Quick Cream of Wheat, 30

Thyme Breakfast Pizza (*Zaatar Manakish*), 42
Yogurt Bowl, 29
Yogurt Spread (*Labne*), 28
Brown Rice with Vermicelli Noodles, 216
brunch recipes
  Breakfast Casserole (*Fatteh*), 38-39
  Cheesy Breakfast Pizza (Cheese *Manakish*), 41-42
  Chicken Liver, 44
  Mediterranean Breakfast Quiche, 39-40
  Shanklish Cheese, 40-41
  Sweet Bread with Dates, 45-46
  Thyme Breakfast Pizza (*Zaatar Manakish*), 42-43
bulgur
  Bulgur Chickpea Pilaf, 119
  Bulgur Tomato Pilaf, 120
  Bulgur with Seasoned Lamb, 118-119
  Lentils and Bulgur Wheat Pilaf, 126

C

cabbage
  Lamb Cabbage Rolls (*Malfouf*), 93-94
  Vegetarian Cabbage Rolls, 213-214
cake recipes, 239
  Date Cake, 243
  Eggless Farina Cake (*Namoura*), 240
  Mediterranean Cheesecakes, 247-248
  Mediterranean Doughnuts, 246
  Olive Oil Cake, 244
  Turmeric Cake (*Sfoof*), 241

Yellow Cake with Jam Topping, 245
Yogurt Cake, 242
cauliflower
  Cauliflower Stew, 83
  Fried Eggplant and Cauliflower Sandwiches, 115
cheese
  Cheesy Breakfast Pizza (Cheese *Manakish*), 41-42
  Fried Cheese, 36
  halloumi cheese, 36
  kashkaval cheese, 42
  Shanklish Cheese, 40-41
  Volcano Feta, 135
cheese recipes
  Cheese Rolls, 144
  Cheesy Breakfast Pizza (Cheese *Manakish*), 41-42
  Mediterranean Grilled Cheese Sandwiches, 114
  Sweet Cheese Rolls, 259
cheesecakes, Mediterranean Cheesecakes, 247-248
chicken recipes
  Barley and Chicken Soup, 76
  Breaded Chicken (Chicken *Escalope*), 95
  Chicken Liver, 44
  Chicken Phyllo Rolls (*Msakhan*), 96
  Chicken Quinoa Pilaf, 97
  Chicken Soup, 69
  Ghallaba Stew
  Jew's Mallow Stew (*Mulukhiya*), 80-81
  main dishes
    Braised Chicken, 194
    Chicken and Potatoes, 193
    Chicken Kefta Kabob, 191-192
    Chicken Roulade, 188-189
    Chicken Shawarma, 186
    Chicken Skewers, 192

Grilled Chicken on the Bone, 195
Mediterranean Meatloaf, 190-191
Roasted Chicken, 189-190
Spiced Chicken and Rice, 187-188
chips, Savory Pita Chips, 149
Chocolate-Dipped Pistachio Sugar Cookies, 231
Chocolate-Peanut Baklava, 234
Cilantro Jalapeño Hummus, 132
Cinnamon Tea, 265
Coconut Puffs, 238
cod, Pan-Seared Cod with Cherry Tomatoes, 200
coffees, Turkish Coffee, 264
cookies
  Chocolate-Dipped Pistachio Sugar Cookies, 231
  Custard Cookie Trifle, 251
  Date Cookies, 229
  Holiday Date Cookies, 230-231
  Jam Cookies, 232
  Pistachio Cookies, 228
couscous
  Sweet and Savory Couscous, 106-107
  Vegetarian Couscous-Stuffed Tomatoes, 208-209
Couscous with Vegetable Stew, 105-106
cucumbers
  Pickled Persian Cucumbers, 220
  Tomato and Cucumber Salad, 53
custards
  Ashta Custard, 258
  Custard Cookie Trifle, 251
  Custard-Filled Pancakes, 256
  Mediterranean Fruit Tart, 261
  Phyllo Custard Pockets, 257

D

Dandelion Greens, 221-222
dates
   Date Balls, 235
   Date Cake, 243
   Date Cookies, 229
   Mascarpone-Stuffed Dates,
    260
   Sweet Bread with Dates, 45-46
dessert recipes, 239
   Ashta Custard, 258
   Baklava, 233
   Chocolate-Dipped Pistachio
    Sugar Cookies, 231
   Chocolate-Peanut Baklava,
    234
   Coconut Puffs, 238
   Custard Cookie Trifle, 251
   Custard-Filled Pancakes, 256
   Date Balls, 235
   Date Cake, 243
   Date Cookies, 229
   Eggless Farina Cake (*Namoura*),
    240
   Fig Bars, 236
   Fig Puffs, 237
   Fried Pancakes, 255
   Fruit Salad, 262
   Halva, 250
   Holiday Date Cookies, 230-231
   Jam Cookies, 232
   Mascarpone-Stuffed Dates,
    260
   Mediterranean Bread Pudding,
    253
   Mediterranean Cheesecakes,
    247-248
   Mediterranean Doughnuts,
    246
   Mediterranean Fruit Tart, 261
   Olive Oil Cake, 244
   Phyllo Custard Pockets, 257
   Pistachio Cookies, 228
   Rice Pudding, 252

   Shredded Phyllo and Sweet
    Cheese Pie, 254
   Simple Syrup, 263
   Sweet Cheese Rolls, 259
   Turmeric Cake (*Sfoof*), 241
   Yellow Cake with Jam
    Topping, 245
   Yogurt Cake, 242
dinner recipes
   beef
    Beef and Potatoes with
     Tahini Sauce, 178-179
    Beef Shawarma, 166
    Beef Shish Kabobs, 170-171
    Dumplings in Yogurt Sauce,
     176-177
    Kefta Kabob, 167
    Kibbeh in a Pan, 169-170
    Kibbeh with Yogurt,
     168-169
    Meat and Rice-Stuffed
     Grape Leaves, 174
    Square Meat Pies, 175
    Stuffed Eggplant Casserole,
     179-180
    Stuffed Squash Casserole,
     177-178
    Tomato and Beef Casserole,
     171-172
   chicken
    Braised Chicken, 194
    Chicken and Potatoes, 193
    Chicken Kefta Kabob,
     191-192
    Chicken Roulade, 188-189
    Chicken Shawarma, 186
    Chicken Skewers, 192
    Grilled Chicken on the
     Bone, 195
    Mediterranean Meatloaf,
     190-191
    Roasted Chicken, 189-190
    Spiced Chicken and Rice,
     187-188

   lamb
    Braised Lamb and
     Tomatoes, 183
    Lamb Chops, 180
    Lamb Meatballs, 182
    Roast Leg of Lamb, 181
    Upside-Down Rice, 172-173
   side dishes
    Brown Rice with Vermicelli
     Noodles, 216
    Dandelion Greens, 221-222
    Green Fava Beans, 218
    Pickled Persian Cucumbers,
     220
    Pickled Turnips, 220-221
    Sautéed Zucchini and
     Mushrooms, 223
    Spiced Meat and Rice, 222
    Spicy Herb Potatoes, 217
    Yellow Rice, 219
   vegetarian
    Vegetarian Baked Spaghetti,
     211-212
    Vegetarian Bowtie Veggie
     Pasta, 207
    Vegetarian Cabbage Rolls,
     213-214
    Vegetarian Couscous-
     Stuffed Tomatoes,
     208-209
    Vegetarian Potato Kibbeh,
     212-213
    Vegetarian Quinoa Pilaf,
     206
    Vegetarian Stuffed Baked
     Potatoes, 209-210
    Vegetarian Stuffed Squash,
     210-211
dips and spreads
   Baba Ganoush, 140
   Cilantro Jalapeño Hummus,
    132
   Eggplant Dip (*Mutabal*),
    137-138
   Hummus with Meat, 131
   Muhammara Spread, 136-137

Olive Tapenade, 138
Roasted Red Pepper and Sun-
Dried Tomato Tapenade, 139
Roasted Red Pepper Hummus,
133
Traditional Hummus, 130
Volcano Feta, 135
White Bean Hummus, 134
disease prevention
Alzheimer's, 5
cancer, 5
depression, 5
heart disease, 4
Type 2 diabetes, 4
dough, Multipurpose Dough, 151
doughnuts, Mediterranean
Doughnuts, 246
dressings, Mediterranean
Dressing, 65
drink recipes
Cinnamon Tea, 265
Turkish Coffee, 264
Dumplings in Yogurt Sauce,
176-177

E

Eggless Farina Cake (*Namoura*),
240
eggplant
Baba Ganoush, 140
Eggplant Casserole, 109-110
Fried Eggplant and
Cauliflower Sandwiches, 115
Stuffed Eggplant Casserole,
179-180
Eggplant Dip (*Mutabal*), 137-138
Eggplant Stew, 79
eggs
Garlic Scrambled Eggs, 31
Herbed Potatoes and Eggs, 35
Holiday Eggs, 32
Mediterranean Breakfast
Quiche, 39-40

Mediterranean Omelet, 33
Potatoes and Eggs Omelet, 34
extra-virgin olive oil, 23

F

Falafel Pita Pockets, 104-105
family involvement, 10
farina, 30
Fatteh (Breakfast Casserole), 38-39
Fattoush Salad, 51
feta, Volcano Feta, 135
Fig Bars, 236
Fig Puffs, 237
Fig Salad, 63
fish
Baked Salmon, 202
Fish and Rice (*Sayadieh*),
198-199
Fish with Tahini Sauce (Fish
Tagine), 98
Pan-Seared Cod with Cherry
Tomatoes, 200
Salmon with Pesto, 201
Spiced Fish, 199-200
Tilapia with a Light Olive
Sauce, 203
Freekeh Pilaf, 121
Freekeh Soup, 75
Fried Cheese, 36
Fried Eggplant and Cauliflower
Sandwiches, 115
Fried Pancakes, 255
fruit recipes
Fruit Salad, 262
Mediterranean Fruit Tart, 261
Ful Mudammas (Breakfast Beans),
43

G

Garlic Sauce, 158
Garlic Scrambled Eggs, 31

Ghallaba Stew, 78
grains, 18-19
grape leaves
Meat and Rice-Stuffed Grape
Leaves, 174
Vegetable Grape Leaves,
108-109
Greek Salad, 60
Green Beans and Tomatoes,
110-111
Green Bean Stew, 84
Green Fava Beans, 218
Green Pea Stew (*Bazella*), 82
Grilled Chicken on the Bone, 195
Grilled Shrimp Sandwiches with
Pesto, 100

H

Halawet el Jibn (Sweet Cheese
Rolls), 259
halloumi cheese, 36
Halva, 250
Harissa (Hot Sauce), 160
health benefits
disease prevention, 4-5
nutritional, 6
weight loss, 5-6
Hearty Brown Lentil Soup, 72-73
Hearty Meat and Potatoes, 89
Herbed Potatoes and Eggs, 35
Holiday Date Cookies, 230-231
Holiday Eggs, 32
Homemade Greek Yogurt, 155
honey, 23
Hot Sauce (*Harissa*), 160
hummus
Cilantro Jalapeño Hummus,
132
Hummus Appetizer Bites, 142
Hummus with Meat, 131
Roasted Red Pepper Hummus,
133

Traditional Hummus, 130
White Bean Hummus, 134

I

ingredient lists, 15-24
cheese and yogurt, 23
eggs, 20
fruits, 16-17
herbs, 22
honey, 23
legumes and nuts, 19-20
meats, 20
olive oil, 22-23
poultry, 20
salt, 22
seafood, 20-21
spices, 22
syrups, 24
vegetables, 17-18
waters, 24
whole grains, 18-19

J

jalapenos, Cilantro Jalapeño
Hummus, 132
Jam Cookies, 232
Jew's Mallow Stew (*Mulukhiya*),
80-81

K

Kabees (Pickled Turnips), 220-221
Kefta Burgers, 87
Kefta Kabob, 167
Kibbeh in a Pan, 169-170
Kibbeh Nayeh (Beef Tartar), 147
Kibbeh with Yogurt, 168-169

Knafe (Shredded Phyllo and Sweet
Cheese Pie), 254
Kusa Mihshi (Beef-Stuffed Squash),
90

L

Labne (Yogurt Spread), 28
Lahme bi Ajeen (Cheeseless Meat
Pizza), 94
lamb recipes
Bulgur with Seasoned Lamb,
118-119
Cheeseless Meat Pizza (*Lahme
bi Ajeen*), 94
Lamb Cabbage Rolls (*Malfouf*),
93-94
Lamb-Stuffed Baked Peppers,
92-93
main dishes
Braised Lamb and
Tomatoes, 183
Lamb Chops, 180
Lamb Meatballs, 182
Roast Leg of Lamb, 181
Upside-Down Rice, 172-173
legumes, 19-20
Lemon Basil Garlic Sauce, 159
Lemon Cilantro Shrimp, 99
Lentil and Swiss Chard Soup, 74
lentils
Hearty Brown Lentil Soup,
72-73
Lentils and Bulgur Wheat
Pilaf, 126
Lentils and Rice, 125
Lentil and Swiss Chard Soup,
74
Lentil Salad, 61
Yellow Lentil Soup, 71-72
liver, Chicken Liver, 44

lunch recipes
beef
Baked Spaghetti with Beef,
88-89
Beef-Stuffed Baked
Potatoes, 91
Beef-Stuffed Squash (*Kusa
Mihshi*), 90
Beefy Pita Sandwiches, 86
Hearty Meat and Potatoes,
89
Kefta Burgers, 87
Bulgur Chickpea Pilaf, 119
Bulgur Tomato Pilaf, 120
Bulgur with Seasoned Lamb,
118-119
chicken
Breaded Chicken (Chicken
Escalope), 95
Chicken Phyllo Rolls
(*Msakhan*), 96
Chicken Quinoa Pilaf, 97
Freekeh Pilaf, 121
lamb
Cheeseless Meat Pizza
(*Lahme bi Ajeen*), 94
Lamb Cabbage Rolls
(*Malfouf*), 93-94
Lamb-Stuffed Baked
Peppers, 92-93
Lentils and Bulgur Wheat
Pilaf, 126
Lentils and Rice, 125
Pumpkin Kibbeh, 123-124
salads
Bean Salad, 62
Fattoush Salad, 51
Fig Salad, 63
Greek Salad, 60
Lentil Salad, 61
Mediterranean Dressing, 65
Mediterranean Garden
Salad, 52
Mediterranean Pasta Salad,
58-59

Mediterranean Potato
Salad, 54-55

Quinoa Salad, 56-57

Roasted Beet Salad, 55-56

Spinach Salad, 59

Tabbouleh Salad, 50

Tomato and Cucumber
Salad, 53

Warm Mediterranean Salad,
57-58

Watermelon Salad, 64

seafood

Basil and Shrimp Quinoa,
102

Fish with Tahini Sauce
(Fish Tagine), 98

Grilled Shrimp Sandwiches
with Pesto, 100

Lemon Cilantro Shrimp, 99

Shrimp and Vegetable Rice,
101

soups, 67

Barley and Chicken Soup,
76

Beef and Vegetable Soup,
68

Chicken Soup, 69

Freekeh Soup, 75

Hearty Brown Lentil Soup,
72-73

Lentil and Swiss Chard
Soup, 74

Pumpkin Soup, 70-71

Yellow Lentil Soup, 71-72

Spiced Tomato No-Bake Pilaf,
122

stews

Cauliflower Stew, 83

Eggplant Stew, 79

Ghallaba Stew, 78

Green Bean Stew, 84

Green Pea Stew (*Bazella*),
82

Jew's Mallow Stew
(*Mulukhiya*), 80-81

Okra Stew (*Bamya*), 81

vegetarian

Couscous with Vegetable
Stew, 105-106

Eggplant Casserole,
109-110

Falafel Pita Pockets,
104-105

Fried Eggplant and
Cauliflower Sandwiches,
115

Green Beans and Tomatoes,
110-111

Macaroni with Yogurt
Sauce, 107-108

Mediterranean Grilled
Cheese Sandwiches, 114

Spanakopita, 112-113

Sweet and Savory
Couscous, 106-107

Vegetable Grape Leaves,
108-109

Zesty Flatbread Pizza, 113

Zucchini Fritters, 111

Zucchini and Brown Rice,
124-125

Kibbeh with Yogurt,
168-169

Meat and Rice-Stuffed
Grape Leaves, 174

Square Meat Pies, 175

Stuffed Eggplant Casserole,
179-180

Stuffed Squash Casserole,
177-178

Tomato and Beef Casserole,
171-172

chicken

Braised Chicken, 194

Chicken and Potatoes, 193

Chicken Kefta Kabob,
191-192

Chicken Roulade, 188-189

Chicken Shawarma, 186

Chicken Skewers, 192

Grilled Chicken on the
Bone, 195

Mediterranean Meatloaf,
190-191

Roasted Chicken, 189-190

Spiced Chicken and Rice,
187-188

lamb

Braised Lamb and
Tomatoes, 183

Lamb Chops, 180

Lamb Meatballs, 182

Roast Leg of Lamb, 181

Upside-Down Rice, 172-173

seafood

Baked Salmon, 202

Fish and Rice (*Sayadieh*),
198-199

Pan-Seared Cod with
Cherry Tomatoes, 200

Salmon with Pesto, 201

Spiced Fish, 199, 200

Tilapia with a Light Olive
Sauce, 203

M

Maamoul (Holiday Date Cookies),
230-231

Macaroni with Yogurt Sauce,
107-108

Macaroons, 238

main dish recipes

beef

Beef and Potatoes with
Tahini Sauce, 178-179

Beef Shawarma, 166

Beef Shish Kabobs, 170-171

Dumplings in Yogurt Sauce,
176-177

Kefta Kabob, 167

Kibbeh in a Pan, 169-170

Makloubeh (Upside-Down Rice),
172-173

Malfouf (Lamb Cabbage Rolls), 93-94

Mascarpone-Stuffed Dates, 260

Meat and Rice-Stuffed Grape Leaves, 174

meatballs, Lamb Meatballs, 182

Meat-Filled Phyllo, 146

meatloaf, Mediterranean Meatloaf, 190-191

Mediterranean Bread Pudding, 253

Mediterranean Breakfast Quiche, 39-40

Mediterranean Cheesecakes, 247-248

Mediterranean diet
    components, 7-8
    dining out considerations, 10
    exercise tips, 9
    family involvement, 10
    food pyramid, 14-15
    health benefits, 4-6
    importance of fresh foods, 8
    lifestyle changes, 10
    planning tips, 10
    stress reduction tips, 9

Mediterranean Doughnuts, 246

Mediterranean Dressing, 65

Mediterranean Fruit Tart, 261

Mediterranean Garden Salad, 52

Mediterranean Grilled Cheese Sandwiches, 114

Mediterranean Meatloaf, 190-191

Mediterranean Omelet, 33

Mediterranean Pasta Salad, 58-59

Mediterranean Potato Salad, 54-55

Moussaka (Eggplant Casserole), 109-110

Msakhan (Chicken Phyllo Rolls), 96

Muhammara Spread, 136-137

Mujaddara Hamra (Lentils and Bulgur Wheat Pilaf), 126

Mujaddara with Rice (Lentils and Rice), 125

Multipurpose Dough, 151

Mulukhiya (Jew's Mallow Stew), 80-81

mushrooms, Sautéed Zucchini and Mushrooms, 223

Mutabal (Eggplant Dip), 137-138

N-O

Namoura (Eggless Farina Cake), 240

nuts, 19-20

Okra Stew (*Bamya*), 81

olive oil
    Olive Oil Cake, 244
    Olive Tapenade, 138

omelets
    Mediterranean Omelet, 33
    Potatoes and Eggs Omelet, 34

P

pancakes
    Custard-Filled Pancakes, 256
    Fried Pancakes, 255

Pan-Seared Cod with Cherry Tomatoes, 200

pantries, stocking, 21-24
    cheese and yogurt, 23
    herbs, 22
    honey, 23
    olive oil, 22-23
    spices, 22
    syrups, 24

pasta recipes
    Baked Spaghetti with Beef, 88-89
    Macaroni with Yogurt Sauce, 107-108
    Mediterranean Pasta Salad, 58-59

Vegetarian Baked Spaghetti, 211-212

Vegetarian Bowtie Veggie Pasta, 207

Vegetarian Couscous-Stuffed Tomatoes, 208-209

peas, Green Pea Stew (*Bazella*), 82

peppers
    Lamb-Stuffed Baked Peppers, 92-93
    Muhammara Spread, 136-137
    Roasted Red Pepper and Sun-Dried Tomato Tapenade, 139
    Roasted Red Pepper Hummus, 133

phyllo
    Meat-Filled Phyllo, 146
    Phyllo Custard Pockets, 257
    Shredded Phyllo and Sweet Cheese Pie, 254

Pickled Persian Cucumbers, 220

Pickled Turnips, 220-221

pies, Shredded Phyllo and Sweet Cheese Pie, 254

pilafs
    Bulgur Chickpea Pilaf, 119
    Bulgur Tomato Pilaf, 120
    Freekeh Pilaf, 121
    Lentils and Bulgur Wheat Pilaf, 126
    Spiced Tomato No-Bake Pilaf, 122

Pistachio Cookies, 228

pita recipes
    Falafel Pita Pockets, 104-105
    Pita Bread, 148-149

pizzas
    Cheeseless Meat Pizza (*Lahme bi Ajeen*), 94
    Cheesy Breakfast Pizza (Cheese *Manakish*), 41-42
    Thyme Breakfast Pizza (*Zaatar Manakish*), 42
    Zesty Flatbread Pizza, 113

potatoes
    Beef and Potatoes with Tahini
        Sauce, 178-179
    Beef-Stuffed Baked Potatoes, 91
    Chicken and Potatoes, 193
    Hearty Meat and Potatoes, 89
    Herbed Potatoes and Eggs, 35
    Mediterranean Potato Salad,
        54-55
    Spicy Herb Potatoes, 217
    Vegetarian Potato Kibbeh,
        212-213
    Vegetarian Stuffed Baked
        Potatoes, 209-210
Potatoes and Eggs Omelet, 34
puddings
    Mediterranean Bread Pudding,
        253
    Rice Pudding, 252
Pumpkin Kibbeh, 123-124
Pumpkin Soup, 70, 71

Q

quiches, Mediterranean Breakfast
    Quiche, 39-40
Quick Cream of Wheat, 30
quinoa, 18
    Basil and Shrimp Quinoa, 102
    Chicken Quinoa Pilaf, 97
    Quinoa Salad, 56-57
    Vegetarian Quinoa Pilaf, 206

R

recipes
    appetizers
        Aromatic Artichokes, 143
        Beef Tartar, 147
        Cheese Rolls, 144
        Hummus Appetizer Bites,
            142
        Meat-Filled Phyllo, 146

        Savory Pita Chips, 149
        Spinach Pies, 145
    breads
        Multipurpose Dough, 151
        Pita Bread, 148-149
        Rosemary Olive Bread, 150
    breakfast, 27
        Fried Cheese, 36
        Garlic Scrambled Eggs, 31
        Herbed Potatoes and Eggs,
            35
        Holiday Eggs, 32
        Mediterranean Omelet, 33
        Potatoes and Eggs Omelet,
            34
        Quick Cream of Wheat, 30
        Yogurt Bowl, 29
        Yogurt Spread (*Labne*), 28
    brunch
        Breakfast Beans (*Ful
            Mudammas*), 43
        Breakfast Casserole (*Fatteh*),
            38-39
        Cheesy Breakfast Pizza
            (Cheese *Manakish*), 41-42
        Chicken Liver, 44
        Mediterranean Breakfast
            Quiche, 39-40
        Shanklish Cheese, 40-41
        Sweet Bread with Dates,
            45-46
        Thyme Breakfast Pizza
            (*Zaatar Manakish*), 42
    desserts, 239
        Ashta Custard, 258
        Baklava, 233
        Chocolate-Dipped
            Pistachio Sugar Cookies,
            231
        Chocolate-Peanut Baklava,
            234
        Coconut Puffs, 238
        Custard Cookie Trifle, 251
        Custard-Filled Pancakes,
            256
        Date Balls, 235

        Date Cake, 243
        Date Cookies, 229
        Eggless Farina Cake
            (*Namoura*), 240
        Fig Bars, 236
        Fig Puffs, 237
        Fried Pancakes, 255
        Fruit Salad, 262
        Halva, 250
        Holiday Date Cookies,
            230-231
        Jam Cookies, 232
        Mascarpone-Stuffed Dates,
            260
        Mediterranean Bread
            Pudding, 253
        Mediterranean
            Cheesecakes, 247-248
        Mediterranean Doughnuts,
            246
        Mediterranean Fruit Tart,
            261
        Olive Oil Cake, 244
        Phyllo Custard Pockets, 257
        Pistachio Cookies, 228
        Rice Pudding, 252
        Shredded Phyllo and Sweet
            Cheese Pie, 254
        Simple Syrup, 263
        Sweet Cheese Rolls, 259
        Turmeric Cake (*Sfoof*), 241
        Yellow Cake with Jam
            Topping, 245
        Yogurt Cake, 242
    dips and spreads
        Baba Ganoush, 140
        Cilantro Jalapeño Hummus,
            132
        Eggplant Dip (*Mutabal*),
            137-138
        Hummus with Meat, 131
        Muhammara Spread,
            136-137
        Olive Tapenade, 138

Roasted Red Pepper and Sun-Dried Tomato Tapenade, 139
Roasted Red Pepper Hummus, 133
Traditional Hummus, 130
Volcano Feta, 135
White Bean Hummus, 134
drinks
Cinnamon Tea, 265
Turkish Coffee, 264
lunch, 67
Baked Spaghetti with Beef, 88-89
Barley and Chicken Soup, 76
Basil and Shrimp Quinoa, 102
Bean Salad, 62
Beef and Vegetable Soup, 68
Beef-Stuffed Baked Potatoes, 91
Beef-Stuffed Squash (*Kusa Mihshi*), 90
Beefy Pita Sandwiches, 86
Breaded Chicken (Chicken Escalope), 95
Bulgur Chickpea Pilaf, 119
Bulgur Tomato Pilaf, 120
Bulgur with Seasoned Lamb, 118-119
Cauliflower Stew, 83
Cheeseless Meat Pizza (*Lahme bi Ajeen*), 94
Chicken Phyllo Rolls (*Msakhan*), 96
Chicken Quinoa Pilaf, 97
Chicken Soup, 69
Couscous with Vegetable Stew, 105-106
Eggplant Casserole, 109-110
Eggplant Stew, 79
Falafel Pita Pockets, 104-105

Fattoush Salad, 51
Fig Salad, 63
Fish with Tahini Sauce (Fish Tagine), 98
Freekeh Pilaf, 121
Freekeh Soup, 75
Fried Eggplant and Cauliflower Sandwiches, 115
Ghallaba Stew, 78
Greek Salad, 60
Green Beans and Tomatoes, 110-111
Green Bean Stew, 84
Green Pea Stew (*Bazella*), 82
Grilled Shrimp Sandwiches with Pesto, 100
Hearty Brown Lentil Soup, 72-73
Hearty Meat and Potatoes, 89
Jew's Mallow Stew (*Mulukhiya*), 80-81
Kefta Burgers, 87
Lamb Cabbage Rolls (*Malfouf*), 93-94
Lamb-Stuffed Baked Peppers, 92-93
Lemon Cilantro Shrimp, 99
Lentil and Swiss Chard Soup, 74
Lentil Salad, 61
Lentils and Bulgur Wheat Pilaf, 126
Lentils and Rice, 125
Macaroni with Yogurt Sauce, 107-108
Mediterranean Dressing, 65
Mediterranean Garden Salad, 52
Mediterranean Grilled Cheese Sandwiches, 114
Mediterranean Pasta Salad, 58-59

Mediterranean Potato Salad, 54-55
Okra Stew (*Bamya*), 81
Pumpkin Kibbeh, 123-124
Pumpkin Soup, 70-71
Quinoa Salad, 56-57
Roasted Beet Salad, 55-56
Shrimp and Vegetable Rice, 101
Spanakopita, 112-113
Spiced Tomato No-Bake Pilaf, 122
Spinach Salad, 59
Sweet and Savory Couscous, 106-107
Tabbouleh Salad, 50
Tomato and Cucumber Salad, 53
Vegetable Grape Leaves, 108-109
Warm Mediterranean Salad, 57-58
Watermelon Salad, 64
Yellow Lentil Soup, 71-72
Zesty Flatbread Pizza, 113
Zucchini and Brown Rice, 124-125
Zucchini Fritters, 111
main dishes
Baked Salmon, 202
Beef and Potatoes with Tahini Sauce, 178-179
Beef Shawarma, 166
Beef Shish Kabobs, 170-171
Braised Chicken, 194
Braised Lamb and Tomatoes, 183
Chicken and Potatoes, 193
Chicken Kefta Kabob, 191-192
Chicken Roulade, 188-189
Chicken Shawarma, 186
Chicken Skewers, 192
Dumplings in Yogurt Sauce, 176-177

Fish and Rice (*Sayadieh*),
198-199
Grilled Chicken on the
Bone, 195
Kefta Kabob, 167
Kibbeh in a Pan, 169-170
Kibbeh with Yogurt,
168-169
Lamb Chops, 180
Lamb Meatballs, 182
Meat and Rice-Stuffed
Grape Leaves, 174
Mediterranean Meatloaf,
190, 191
Pan-Seared Cod with
Cherry Tomatoes, 200
Roasted Chicken, 189-190
Roast Leg of Lamb, 181
Salmon with Pesto, 201
Spiced Chicken and Rice,
187-188
Spiced Fish, 199-200
Square Meat Pies, 175
Stuffed Eggplant Casserole,
179-180
Stuffed Squash Casserole,
177-178
Tilapia with a Light Olive
Sauce, 203
Tomato and Beef Casserole,
171-172
Upside-Down Rice, 172-173
sauces
Garlic Sauce, 158
Homemade Greek Yogurt,
155
Hot Sauce (*Harissa*), 160
Lemon Basil Garlic Sauce,
159
Tahini Paste, 156
Tahini Sauce, 157
Tzatziki Sauce, 154
side dishes
Brown Rice with Vermicelli
Noodles, 216
Dandelion Greens, 221-222

Green Fava Beans, 218
Pickled Persian Cucumbers,
220
Pickled Turnips, 220-221
Sautéed Zucchini and
Mushrooms, 223
Spiced Meat and Rice, 222
Spicy Herb Potatoes, 217
Yellow Rice, 219
spices
Seven Spice Mix, 162
Zaatar, 161
vegetarian
Vegetarian Baked Spaghetti,
211-212
Vegetarian Bowtie Veggie
Pasta, 207
Vegetarian Cabbage Rolls,
213-214
Vegetarian Couscous-
Stuffed Tomatoes,
208-209
Vegetarian Potato Kibbeh,
212-213
Vegetarian Quinoa Pilaf,
206
Vegetarian Stuffed Baked
Potatoes, 209-210
Vegetarian Stuffed Squash,
210-211
rice
Brown Rice with Vermicelli
Noodles, 216
Fish and Rice (*Sayadieh*),
198-199
Lentils and Rice, 125
Shrimp and Vegetable Rice, 101
Spiced Chicken and Rice,
187-188
Spiced Meat and Rice, 222
Upside-Down Rice, 172-173
Yellow Rice, 219
Zucchini and Brown Rice,
124-125
Rice Pudding, 252
Roasted Beet Salad, 55-56

Roasted Chicken, 189-190
Roasted Red Pepper and Sun-
Dried Tomato Tapenade, 139
Roasted Red Pepper Hummus, 133
Roast Leg of Lamb, 181
Rosemary Olive Bread, 150

S

salad recipes
Bean Salad, 62
Fattoush Salad, 51
Fig Salad, 63
Greek Salad, 60
Lentil Salad, 61
Mediterranean Dressing, 65
Mediterranean Garden Salad,
52
Mediterranean Pasta Salad,
58-59
Mediterranean Potato Salad,
54-55
Quinoa Salad, 56-57
Roasted Beet Salad, 55-56
Spinach Salad, 59
Tabbouleh Salad, 50
Tomato and Cucumber Salad,
53
Warm Mediterranean Salad,
57-58
Watermelon Salad, 64
salmon
Baked Salmon, 202
Salmon with Pesto, 201
Samboosek (Meat-Filled Phyllo), 146
sandwiches
Beefy Pita Sandwiches, 86
Fried Eggplant and
Cauliflower Sandwiches, 115
Grilled Shrimp Sandwiches
with Pesto, 100
Kefta Burgers, 87
Mediterranean Grilled Cheese
Sandwiches, 114

sauce recipes
  Garlic Sauce, 158
  Homemade Greek Yogurt, 155
  Hot Sauce (*Harissa*), 160
  Lemon Basil Garlic Sauce, 159
  Tahini Paste, 156
  Tahini Sauce, 157
  Tzatziki Sauce, 154
Sautéed Zucchini and
  Mushrooms, 223
Savory Pita Chips, 149
Sayadieh (Fish and Rice), 198-199
seafood recipes
  Baked Salmon, 202
  Basil and Shrimp Quinoa, 102
  Fish and Rice (*Sayadieh*),
    198-199
  Fish with Tahini Sauce (Fish
    Tagine), 98
  Grilled Shrimp Sandwiches
    with Pesto, 100
  Lemon Cilantro Shrimp, 99
  Pan-Seared Cod with Cherry
    Tomatoes, 200
  Salmon with Pesto, 201
  Shrimp and Vegetable Rice,
    101
  Spiced Fish, 199-200
  Tilapia with a Light Olive
    Sauce, 203
Seven Spice Mix, 162
Sfeeha (Square Meat Pies), 175
Sfoof (Turmeric Cake), 241
Shaabiyat (Phyllo Custard
  Pockets), 257
Shanklish Cheese, 40, 41
Shish Tawook (Chicken Skewers),
  192
Shredded Phyllo and Sweet
  Cheese Pie, 254
Shrimp and Vegetable Rice, 101
shrimp recipes
  Basil and Shrimp Quinoa, 102
  Grilled Shrimp Sandwiches
    with Pesto, 100
  Lemon Cilantro Shrimp, 99

Shrimp and Vegetable Rice,
  101
side dish recipes
  Brown Rice with Vermicelli
    Noodles, 216
  Dandelion Greens, 221-222
  Green Fava Beans, 218
  Pickled Persian Cucumbers,
    220
  Pickled Turnips, 220-221
  Sautéed Zucchini and
    Mushrooms, 223
  Spiced Meat and Rice, 222
  Spicy Herb Potatoes, 217
  Yellow Rice, 219
Simple Syrup, 263
snacks
  appetizers
    Aromatic Artichokes, 143
    Beef Tartar, 147
    Cheese Rolls, 144
    Hummus Appetizer Bites,
      142
    Meat-Filled Phyllo, 146
    Savory Pita Chips, 149
    Spinach Pies, 145
  breads
    Multipurpose Dough, 151
    Pita Bread, 148-149
    Rosemary Olive Bread, 150
  dips and spreads
    Baba Ganoush, 140
    Cilantro Jalapeño Hummus,
      132
    Eggplant Dip (*Mutabal*),
      137-138
    Hummus with Meat, 131
    Muhammara Spread,
      136-137
    Olive Tapenade, 138
    Roasted Red Pepper and
      Sun-Dried Tomato
      Tapenade, 139
    Roasted Red Pepper
      Hummus, 133
    Traditional Hummus, 130

    Volcano Feta, 135
    White Bean Hummus, 134
soup recipes, 67. *See also* stew
  recipes
  Barley and Chicken Soup, 76
  Beef and Vegetable Soup, 68
  Chicken Soup, 69
  Freekeh Soup, 75
  Hearty Brown Lentil Soup,
    72-73
  Lentil and Swiss Chard Soup,
    74
  Pumpkin Soup, 70-71
  Yellow Lentil Soup, 71-72
spaghetti, Vegetarian Baked
  Spaghetti, 211-212
Spanakopita, 112-113
Spiced Chicken and Rice, 187-188
Spiced Fish, 199-200
Spiced Meat and Rice, 222
Spiced Tomato No-Bake Pilaf,
  122
spices
  Seven Spice Mix, 162
  seven spices, 34
  stocking pantries, 22
  Zaatar, 161
spinach
  Spanakopita, 112-113
  Spinach Pies, 145
  Spinach Salad, 59
Square Meat Pies, 175
squash
  Beef-Stuffed Squash (*Kusa
    Mihshi*), 90
  Stuffed Squash Casserole,
    177-178
  Vegetarian Stuffed Squash,
    210-211
stew recipes. *See also* soup recipes
  Cauliflower Stew, 83
  Couscous with Vegetable Stew,
    105-106
  Eggplant Stew, 79
  Ghallaba Stew, 78
  Green Bean Stew, 84

Green Pea Stew (*Bazella*), 82
Jew's Mallow Stew (*Mulukhiya*),
    80-81
Okra Stew (*Bamya*), 81
stocking pantries, 21-24
Stuffed Eggplant Casserole,
    179-180
Stuffed Squash Casserole, 177-178
Sweet and Savory Couscous,
    106-107
Sweet Bread with Dates, 45-46
Sweet Cheese Rolls, 259

T

Tabbouleh Salad, 50
Tahini Paste, 156
Tahini Sauce, 157
tapenades
    Olive Tapenade, 138
    Roasted Red Pepper and Sun-
        Dried Tomato Tapenade, 139
teas, Cinnamon Tea, 265
Thyme Breakfast Pizza (*Zaatar
    Manakish*), 42
Tilapia with a Light Olive Sauce,
    203
Tomato and Beef Casserole,
    171-172
Tomato and Cucumber Salad, 53
tomatoes
    Braised Lamb and Tomatoes,
        183
    Bulgur Tomato Pilaf, 120
    Green Beans and Tomatoes,
        110-111
    Roasted Red Pepper and Sun-
        Dried Tomato Tapenade, 139
    Spiced Tomato No-Bake Pilaf,
        122
    Vegetarian Couscous-Stuffed
        Tomatoes, 208-209
Traditional Hummus, 130
Turkish Coffee, 264

Turmeric Cake (*Sfoof*), 241
turnips, Pickled Turnips, 220-221
Tzatziki Sauce, 154

V

Vegetable Grape Leaves, 108-109
vegetarian recipes
    dinner
        Vegetarian Baked Spaghetti,
            211-212
        Vegetarian Bowtie Veggie
            Pasta, 207
        Vegetarian Cabbage Rolls,
            213-214
        Vegetarian Couscous-
            Stuffed Tomatoes,
            208-209
        Vegetarian Potato Kibbeh,
            212-213
        Vegetarian Quinoa Pilaf,
            206
        Vegetarian Stuffed Baked
            Potatoes, 209-210
        Vegetarian Stuffed Squash,
            210-211
    lunch
        Couscous with Vegetable
            Stew, 105-106
        Eggplant Casserole,
            109-110
        Falafel Pita Pockets,
            104-105
        Fried Eggplant and
            Cauliflower Sandwiches,
            115
        Green Beans and Tomatoes,
            110-111
        Macaroni with Yogurt
            Sauce, 107-108
        Mediterranean Grilled
            Cheese Sandwiches, 114
        Spanakopita, 112-113
        Sweet and Savory

Couscous, 106-107
    Vegetable Grape Leaves,
        108-109
    Zesty Flatbread Pizza, 113
    Zucchini Fritters, 111
Volcano Feta, 135

W-X-Y-Z

Warm Mediterranean Salad,
    57-58
Watermelon Salad, 64
water, 24
White Bean Hummus, 134
whole grains, 18-19

Yellow Cake with Jam Topping,
    245
Yellow Lentil Soup, 71-72
Yellow Rice, 219
yogurt
    Dumplings in Yogurt Sauce,
        176-177
    Homemade Greek Yogurt, 155
    Kibbeh with Yogurt, 168-169
    Macaroni with Yogurt Sauce,
        107-108
    Yogurt Bowl, 29
    Yogurt Cake, 242
    Yogurt Spread (*Labne*), 28

Zaatar, 161
Zaatar Manakish (Thyme
    Breakfast Pizza), 42
Zesty Flatbread Pizza, 113
zucchini
    Sautéed Zucchini and
        Mushrooms, 223
    Zucchini and Brown Rice, 124,
        125
    Zucchini Fritters, 111